Wound Care Nursing

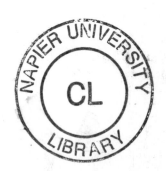

WOUND CARE NURSING

A Patient-centred Approach

Sue Bale

Director of Nursing Research

and

Vanessa Jones

Educational Facilitator

Wound Healing Unit
University of Wales College of Medicine
Cardiff, UK

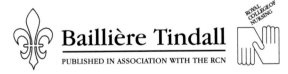

Baillière Tindall

PUBLISHED IN ASSOCIATION WITH THE RCN

London   Philadelphia   Toronto   Sydney   Tokyo

Baillière Tindall 24–28 Oval Road,
London NW1 7DX, UK

The Curtis Center
Independence Square West
Philadelphia, PA 19106–3399, USA

Harcourt Brace & Company
55 Horner Avenue
Toronto, Ontario M8Z 4X6, Canada

Harcourt Brace & Company, Australia
30–52 Smidmore Street
Marrickville, NSW 2204, Australia

Harcourt Brace & Company, Japan
Ichibancho Central Building,
22-1 Ichibancho
Chiyoda-ku, Tokyo 102, Japan

A catalogue record for this book is available from the
British Library

ISBN 0–7020–1870–8

This book is printed on acid-free paper

Cover illustration courtesy of Sam Tanner, Photographer

Typeset by J&L Composition Ltd, Filey, North Yorkshire
Printed and bound in Hong Kong by Dah Hua Printing Press Co., Ltd

CONTENTS

Preface

For many years, wound management had a low profile in both the nursing and medical worlds, with little awareness of issues related to the care of patients with wounds and wound problems.

In the early 1980s, a gradual change in attitudes occurred. This has since snowballed and there are now several societies and associations, journals, books and conferences dedicated solely to the problems of managing patients with wounds. Many of the currently available books on wound management are designed for the post-registered nurse who has some experience in this field of nursing and they assume a level of knowledge accordingly.

This book aims to be different. It attempts to link the holistic approach to wound care with nursing theory. For many nurses in clinical practice, nursing theory is unfamiliar and has little apparent relevance to their daily practice. The new approach this book offers is to use the nursing process and nursing models to help the reader see how to apply *theory to practice*. The book is designed to meet the needs of the student new to wound care nursing. By developing the skills of assessment, planning, management and evaluation of care, the reader can focus on the patient and their wound-related problems. This new approach helps the student nurse and non-specialist nurses in community and hospital practice place wound care in the context of nursing generally. Wound care can therefore become part of the evaluation of the care of the patient as a whole as well as in relation to the wound itself.

The material contained in this book is based on research-based evidence and referenced extensively. Suggested further reading is provided for those readers who wish to pursue topics of interest in more depth. The use of analysis from the reader and case study material provides the student with realism. Although each chapter contains worked examples of care plans, the student also has the opportunity to work through and formulate care plans of their own using a model of their own choosing. The interactive style of the book is designed to encourage the reader to participate and encourages analytical and problem solving skills.

It can also be used by the experienced wound care practitioner to enhance their own practice and help them with their own responsibilities of preceptorship with students. Nurses working and studying in the community will find that a significant proportion of the examples are community-based and the majority of information is relevant to wound care regardless of setting. This is deliberate as most patients will spend most of their healing time in the community.

The book is divided into three sections, reflecting the stages of the nursing process:

Part 1. This section deals with assessment and planning of care and provides the theoretical basis required for the student to proceed to the next section.
Part 2. The chapters in Part 2 are linked to significant stages in the life-cycle, commencing with the baby and young child, and moving through teenage years to young, middle and mature adulthood, and concluding with two chapters devoted to the important stage of the elderly years. This gives the reader an insight into the variety and range of problems that affect and influence patients. Management interventions are illustrated with realistic case studies and the theories which have been outlined in Part 1 are clearly related to the clinical situation.
Part 3. This final section discusses methods of evaluating care, and provides a structured framework for this process.

We hope that by reading this book and working through the Practice Points provided, nurses will be able to relate each chapter to their own experience, so broadening their knowledge base and enhancing their status as professionals.

Sue Bale
Vanessa Jones

Authors' note

Please note: all names used in the Case Studies are fictitious.

Publisher's Acknowledgements

Figures 1.5, 1.22, 6.10, Table 1.4 reproduced with kind permission of *Journal of Wound Care*, London.

Figures 1.8, 1.9, reproduced with kind permission of Dr C Lawrence, Wound Healing Research Unit, Cardiff.

Figure 2.2, from Chapman (1985) *Theory of Nursing; Practical Application* published by Harper & Row. Reproduced with kind permission from Christine Chapman.

Figure 4.6, from Settle (1986) *Burns—The First 5 Days*, reproduced by kind permission of Smith & Nephew Healthcare Ltd, Hull.

Figure 5.1, reproduced with kind permission of Jan Olsens, Burns Unit, Morriston Hospital.

Figure 6.11, reproduced from Beischer & Mackay (1986) *Obstetrics and the Newborn* 2/e published by Baillière Tindall, London.

Table 7.2, from Alexander *et al.* (eds) (1994), *Nursing Practice, Hospital and Home—The Adult*. Reproduced by kind permission of Churchill Livingstone, Edinburgh.

Figure 8.1, from Compendium of Health Statistics 8th Edition, (1992), reproduced with kind permission of Office of Health Economics, London.

Table 8.3, The Waterlow Pressure Sore Prevention/Treatment Policy Care, reproduced with kind permission of JA Waterlow.

Figure 9.7, Doppler Ankle Pressure Index (API) Guide, reproduced with kind permission of HNE Diagnostics, Cardiff.

Figure 10.1, from J Kundin *et al.*, (1989) *A New Way to Size Up a Wound*. Reproduced with kind permission of the American Journal of Nursing Company.

Appendix from Harding, K & Jones V, Wound Management—Good Practice Guidelines, published by *Journal of Wound Care*, London. Reproduced with kind permission of *Journal of Wound Care*, London.

All clinical pictures other than those listed above were kindly supplied by Dr KG Harding, Wound Healing Research Unit, Cardiff.

ASSESSMENT AND PLANNING

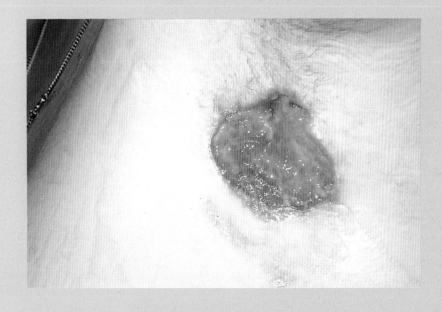

Assessing the Normal and Abnormal

Key issues

This chapter introduces the reader to the factors that need to be considered in order to perform a full assessment. The following areas are covered:

Assessment of the Individual to Include

- Normal stages of healing
- Abnormalities of healing
- Wounds healing by primary and secondary intention

Factors that Affect Healing

- Intrinsic
- Extrinsic

Assessment of the Wound

- Sutured/granulating
- Shape and size
- Recognition of infection

Assessment of the Environment

- Hospital or community based

Case Study 1.1
Adeno-carcinoma of the rectum

Mr David Simons, a 52-year-old-man, had previously been admitted to hospital with a history of rectal bleeding, intermittent diarrhoea and lower abdominal colic.

He was diagnosed as having an invasive adenocarcinoma of the rectum and treated with radiotherapy and chemotherapy. Surgery was not planned at that stage as he was still opening his bowels without difficulty, and it was decided to reassess the patient after treatment.

Prior to the initial consultation David had lost 45 kg in weight and had separated from his wife, who lived with their eight children in a two-bedroomed flat, while he lived in a YMCA hostel.

Following treatment he was due to return some weeks later with a view to surgery for a defunctioning colostomy, but was admitted in the interim period with a 1-week history of a swollen, painful right leg.

David was cachectic, with pyrexia (37.5 °C); blood tests revealed a haemoglobin level of 7.9 g/dl and a serum albumin concentration of 18 g/l. His leg was swollen from hip to foot, especially over the lateral aspect of his thigh, where there was also evidence of surgical emphysema.

Emergency surgery revealed that the colon had perforated owing to the advancing tumour, and the colonic contents had caused surgical emphysema in the tissue of the right leg. Infection had spread rapidly, causing necrotizing fasciitis and therefore gross destruction of the tissue and muscle of the pelvis, hip and thigh region.

Necrotic tissue
the death of previously viable tissue

David was taken to theatre three times over the following 5 days for excision and debridement of the **necrotic tissue** and formation of a colostomy. The wounds that resulted from this surgical intervention (Figure 1.1) were:

i) large cavity down to muscle fascia and penetrating into the pelvic cavity on the lateral aspect of the hip, drained with a size 36 sump drain tube

ii) cavity on the medial aspect of the thigh

iii) 10 cm × 6 cm cavity on the lateral calf

iv) 3 cm × 2 cm cavity on the dorsum of the foot

Thought unlikely to survive the initial surgery, post-operatively David became depressed and withdrawn, was in a great deal of pain especially at dressing changes, and was unable to tolerate any substantial diet.

Figure 1.1
David Simons following emergency surgery.

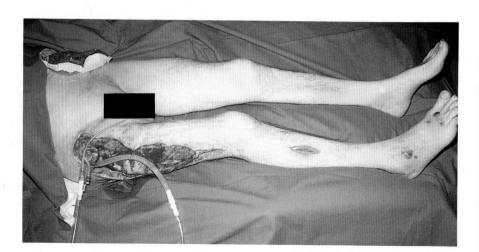

Introduction

The problems described in Case Study 1.1 are not typical of those facing nurses in their day-to-day work. Mr Simon's case is, however, an excellent example of the many factors that can complicate the normal process of healing. The effective management of patients with wounds and wound problems depends upon the nurse taking a systematic, logical, holistic approach. This organized approach consists of assessment of the individual, the wound and the environment (Figure 1.2).

Assessment of the Individual

Assessment of the overall health of the individual will highlight factors that may impair the normal healing process. However, before an understanding of these factors can be appreciated it is important that the nurse is knowledgeable about the normal healing process.

Normal Wound Healing

Wound healing can be divided into its constituent phases, usually described as **haemostasis**, **inflammation**, **proliferation** and **maturation** (Figure 1.3).

It should be remembered that these processes take place concurrently and do not always follow one another in an orderly sequence.

Figure 1.2   *A holistic approach to wound assessment.*

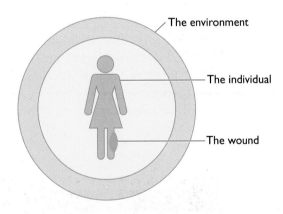

The environment

The individual

The wound

Figure 1.3   *The wound healing process. Although for convenience the wound healing process is considered here in four phases, it is important to remember that healing is a dynamic, ongoing process. It begins at day 0 with initial wounding but can continue for several years.*

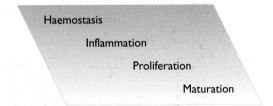

Haemostasis

Inflammation

Proliferation

Maturation

Haemostasis

Haemostasis
the process of stopping bleeding

Extravasation
a discharge or escape of blood or fluid from a vessel in the tissues

Leucocytes
the colourless blood corpuscle which protects the body against micro-organisms

Following cutaneous injury to blood vessels and endothelial cells, blood **extravasation** into the skin initiates platelet activation and blood coagulation. Activated platelets facilitate wound repair by promoting haemostasis (Figure 1.4), blood constriction and new tissue formation (Centre for Medical Education 1992). A short period of vasoconstriction occurs owing to the release of chemical mediators such as histamine, serotonin and adenosine triphosphate (ATP). Most of these mediators act as chemoattractants to circulating **leucocytes**, bringing them to the injured area.

Following initial vasoconstriction the inflammatory process begins with the release of prostaglandins and activated complement proteins causing widespread vasodilation and inflammation (Silver 1994).

Inflammatory Phase

Inflammation
the initial response to tissue injury

Macrophage
any of the large, mononuclear, phagocytotic cells

Angiogenesis
the process of new blood vessel formation

Endothelium
the layer of epithelial cells that line the cavities of the heart, the blood and lymph vessels and the serous cavities of the body

With an increase in blood there is increased capillary permeability thus allowing plasma to leak into the surrounding tissue producing inflammatory exudate. Neutrophils and monocytes are attracted to the wound by a variety of chemotactic factors. Both arrive at the site of injury in a quiescent state and require activation (Rigby 1992). Following activation neutrophils rid the wound of contaminating bacteria. Monocytes undergo a phenotypic change to the activated **macrophage** which produces growth factors that either start, accelerate or modify the healing process. They also produce cytokines that act as messengers between macrophages and other cells.

Macrophages also phagocytose and kill pathogenic organisms and scavenge tissue debris, including old neutrophils (Whitby 1995).

The formation of new blood vessels occurs with the release of **angiogenic** growth factors which stimulate **endothelium** to divide and direct the growth of new blood vessels (Silver 1994).

Figure 1.4
Haemostasis.

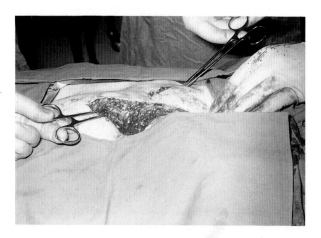

Proliferative Phase

Proliferation
the growth or reproduction of tissue as part of the healing process

Fibroblast
an immature collagen-producing cell of connective tissue

Collagen
the main protein constituent of white fibrous tissue

Granulation tissue
the new tissue formed during the proliferative phase of wound healing

Proline
a cyclic amino acid occurring in proteins

Epithelialization
the growth of epithelium over a denuded wound surface

Myofibroblast
a differentiated fibroblast containing the ultra-structural features of a fibroblast and a smooth muscle cell and containing actin-rich microfilaments

Figure 1.5 *Healthy granulation tissue on the wound bed of a pilonidal sinus excision.*

The formation of new connective tissue (granulation tissue) is dependent on the formation of these new blood vessels in the wound (Figure 1.5). Initially the wound is hypoxic and lacking in nutrients, but as capillary loops are formed the environment becomes oxygenated (Silver 1994).

The macrophages next recruit a new type of cell, the **fibroblast**, which produces a network of **collagen** surrounding the neovasculature of the wound. Fibroblasts also produce proteoglycans, a glue-like ground substance which fills the tissue space, coating and binding fibres together giving them greater flexibility, and fibronectin, which forms the framework for tissue by holding collagen and cells together while attaching them to the ground substance. **Granulation tissue** formation begins after a lag period of several days, but already by day 5 large numbers of fibroblasts have been recruited into the area by the macrophages, and the synthesis of collagen and ground substance has begun. In order to synthesize collagen properly, fibroblasts depend on oxygen and nutrients supplied by the newly forming blood vessel system. In particular, vitamin C (ascorbic acid) acts as a coenzyme for the hydroxylation of **proline** in collagen to hydroxyproline. Collagen formed without adequate vitamin C is weaker as inadequate cross-linking of fibres reduces the tensile quality of the healed wound (Rigby 1992).

During proliferation two other processes are taking place simultaneously — epithelialization and contraction. **Epithelialization** resurfaces the wound by regenerating epithelium. Where damage is extensive and involves deep dermal tissue loss, regeneration occurs from the wound margins. Where there is superficial skin loss, remnants of hair follicles will act as islands of regenerating epithelium. Migration across the wound surface continues until other epithelial cells are met. The migration then ceases, a complex process known as contact inhibition. Wound contraction decreases the size of the wound, a process largely due to the work of the **myofibro-**

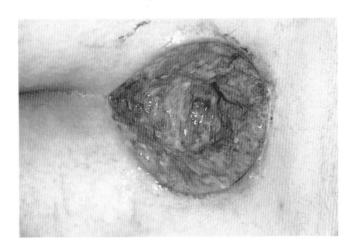

blast. Myofibroblasts under the influence of inflammatory mediators reduce the surface area of the wound before cellular proliferation takes place. The myofibroblast is a differentiated fibroblast containing actin and myosin fibrils (Whitby 1995). Once an open cavity has filled with new granulation tissue and epithelialization has occurred, the proliferative phase of healing stops.

Maturation Phase

Maturation
a phase in wound healing where scar tissue is remodelled

The final stage of healing begins roughly 3 weeks after injury and is a process of remodelling of the collagen fibres laid down during the proliferation phase (Figure 1.6).

During the maturation phase, type III collagen, a soft gelatinous collagen, is gradually replaced with stronger, more highly organized collagen. Differentiation of collagen is a dynamic process, and although it commences predominantly during maturation, may continue indefinitely.

The balance between collagen breakdown and production is a finely balanced process and unless maintained can result in delayed or inadequate healing. Once established, the amount of collagen bed does not alter, just the type and formation within the wound. Type III collagen is removed by collagenases and synthesis of type I collagen occurs, laid down in a more orderly network, fashioned along the lines of tension.

The process of remodelling continues with the fibroblasts migrating from the wound site, and there is rationalization of the numerous blood vessels resulting in shrinking, thinning and paling of the scar.

Healing by Primary Intention

Suture
a stitch or series of stitches made to secure opposition of the edges of a surgical or traumatic wound

Healing by primary intention occurs following a clean surgical incision where the edges of the wound are closely approximated, thus eliminating dead space. There is a minimal formation of granulation tissue, and once the wound has healed only a thin seam remains. All the above phases of wound healing occur, but following the initial inflammatory response wound contraction has a minor role, and epithelium migrates over the **suture** line to restore tissue integrity (Whitby 1995).

Figure 1.6 *A healed pilonidal sinus excision in the maturation phase.*

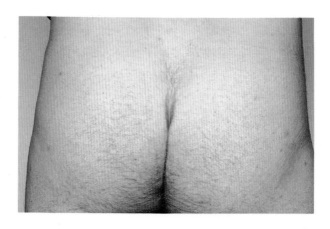

Figure 1.7 *An axillary wound healing by secondary intention.*

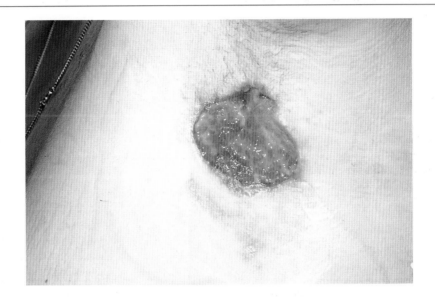

Healing by Secondary Intention

Healing by secondary intention (Figure 1.7) occurs in wounds where there is a large tissue defect. The wound must heal by formation of granulation tissue and wound contraction, resulting in dense, fibrous scar tissue. Generally these wounds take longer to heal because of the large amounts of granulation tissue required. The proliferative and maturation phases are longer than in wounds healing by primary intention.

Healing by Third Intention

Infection
invasion of micro-organisms in body fluids or tissues

Where the presence of **infection** or a foreign body is suspected a wound may be left open to commence healing by granulation until the presenting problem has been resolved. The wound edges are then approximated and healing by primary intention can proceed.

Abnormal Wound Healing

Unfortunately, failure to achieve adequate healing is relatively common. Abnormalities of wound healing are described below.

Keloids

Keloid
a type of scar which is often red and prominent

Keloids result from the formation of large amounts of scar tissue around the site of the wound (Figure 1.8). This is due to an increase in collagen synthesis and lysis and is also thought to be linked to the melanocyte stimulating hormone, as it is very common in people with pigmented skin. Often these scars are larger than the wound itself, and even following excision the scar is likely to recur.

Hypertrophic Scars

Hypertrophic
an increase in volume of tissue produced by enlargement of existing cells

Keloid and **hypertrophic** scars are often similar, but hypertrophic scars (Figure 1.9) tend to follow the line of the incision and are more common in the young. Careful placing of incisions along Langer's lines (Centre for Medical Education 1992) and fine suture material can often avoid excessive scar formation.

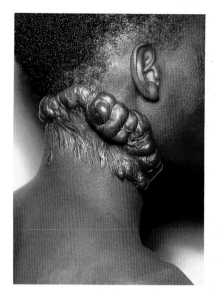

Figure 1.8 *Keloid scarring.*

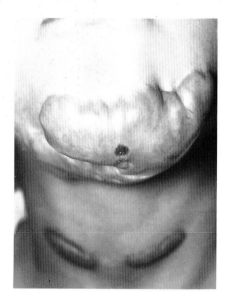

Figure 1.9 *Hypertrophic scarring.*

Atrophic Scars

Atrophic scars are weak and thin and resemble stretch marks. Although there is little to explain why they occur (as with the other abnormalities), they are more common in certain individuals than others.

Contractures

Contractures
abnormal shortening of muscle or scar tissue rendering the muscle highly resistant to stretching

Contractures occur when there is excessive wound contraction and is greatest in skin not tethered to underlying deep fascia or other structures. Again, it is not fully understood why this occurs in some people and not others, but it is important when planning surgical procedures to consider the effect of contraction — especially in areas around the joints.

Dehiscence

Dehiscence
a splitting open or separation of the layers of a surgically closed wound

Haematoma
a localized collection of blood which can form in an organ, space or tissue

Dehiscence occurs when the wound has failed to develop sufficient strength to withstand forces placed upon it. It occurs most commonly 5–10 days post-operatively, although it can occur up to a month after surgery.

The patient often presents with pyrexia and wound discharge of sero-sanguineous fluid. The risk is always increased by localized wound infection, **haematoma** formation or excessive tension placed on the wound by coughing.

Incisional hernia

Incisional hernias (Figure 1.10) can develop months or even years following surgery, and represent failure of part of the scar to develop sufficient strength. They occur more often in infected wounds and in the obese.

Figure 1.10 *An incisional hernia.*

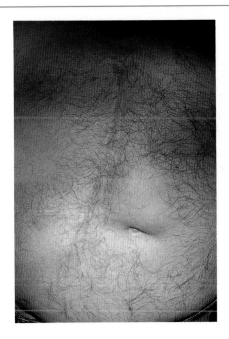

Malignant changes

Any long-standing ulcer may undergo malignant changes to form a squamous cell carcinoma. Although the precise mechanism is not known, with such a rapid turnover of cells in any wound it is important that the practitioner should bear in mind the possibility of malignancy.

Any wound that has an unusual appearance or fails to heal over a long period should be investigated.

Factors Affecting Wound Healing

Many abnormalities of wound healing can be prevented by careful assessment before, during and after surgery. Identification and treatment of local and systemic conditions can also optimize the patient's care.

Key factors adversely affecting wound healing are listed in Table 1.1. Some such factors may be treatable or preventable, and following identification of the problem, treatment should be given. However, where this is not possible,

Table 1.1 *Factors adversely affecting the healing process*

Intrinsic factors	Extrinsic factors
Age	Poor surgical technique
Disease processes/metabolic	Poor wound care
Psychological status	Malnutrition
Body image	Fluid balance
	Smoking
	Drug therapies
	Radiotherapy

factors known to affect healing should be documented and the possibility of delayed healing be planned for.

Intrinsic Factors

Age

With advancing age the metabolic processes — including the wound healing process — begin to slow down, so prolonging the healing phase. Tensile wound strength is often affected owing to reduced collagen production and poor circulation associated with old age.

Disease

A whole range of disease processes that adversely affect metabolism are also likely to delay or prevent wound healing:

Arteriosclerosis
a group of diseases
characterized by thickening
and loss of the elasticity of
the arterial walls

- Anaemia
- **Arteriosclerosis**
- Cancer
- Cardiovascular disorders
- Diabetes
- Immune disorders
- Inflammatory diseases
- Jaundice, liver failure
- Rheumatoid arthritis
- Uraemia

In some vulnerable groups of patients, especially the elderly, several disease processes may be present in one individual at the same time.

Psychological factors

The association between the psychological and the physical well-being of individuals is now recognized as important. Psychological problems can have an adverse effect on the health of patients. Stress and anxiety in particular can affect the immune system (Maier and Laudenslager 1985). Stress hormones especially are linked with the immune sympathetic and central nervous systems (Deitch and Bridges 1987).

Linked with stress are sleep disturbances. Sleep is thought to be essential for healing and tissue repair. Sleep encourages anabolism and, as wounded healing includes anabolic processes, it has been suggested that healing is promoted by rest and sleep (Adam and Oswald 1983).

Body image

An individual's perception of his or her own appearance constitutes the concept of body image and is an important, integral aspect of the self. Either through surgery or by developing a chronic wound, the individual's body image is changed or altered. Altered body image can have dramatic negative effects, especially when disfiguring surgery has been performed such as mastectomy, stoma formation or the amputation of a limb. The grieving process is associated with this negative alteration in body image (Dealey 1994).

Extrinsic Factors

Poor surgical technique

The most common problem associated with poor surgical technique is haematoma formation, caused by rough handling of tissues and by inappropriate use of diathermy or wound drains. This can lead to the presence of a dead space, encouraging wound infection as the haematoma is broken down.

Tissues can also be damaged by poor suturing technique, when sutures are inserted too tightly.

Poor wound care

Wound healing may be impeded by poor dressing technique or the inappropriate use of a dressing material or antiseptic solution. These problems can be avoided by careful assessment by a practitioner with a sound knowledge and understanding of the principles of managing patients with wounds.

Malnutrition

The healthy process requires a ready and adequate supply of nutrients. Malnutrition can result in delays in wound healing, resulting in weak, poor-quality scars (Pinchcofsky-Devin 1994).

Trace element deficiency

- Zinc is an essential cofactor for the enzymatic activity of 200 or more enzymes, including protein synthesis (McLaren 1992), and zinc deficiency has long been known to impair wound healing. Patients who are zinc deficient have reduced rates of epithelialization, decreased wound strength and reduced collagen synthesis (Pinchcofsky-Devin 1994).
- Copper is needed for the cross-linkage of collagen. Although rare, copper deficiency reduces the activity of an enzyme, lysyl oxidase, essential in collagen formation. Patients receiving long-term total parenteral nutrition and malabsorption syndrome are most at risk (McLaren 1992).
- Iron – collagen synthesis relies on iron as it is an essential cofactor for both lysyl and prolyl hydroxylase. In addition, anaemia may impair healing through reducing oxygen transportation (McLaren 1992).

Protein-energy malnutrition

The problem of malnutrition occurs not only in impoverished countries, but also exists in the UK today. Hospital patients can be at risk of protein-energy

Table 1.2 *Patients at risk of hospital-induced protein-energy malnutrition*

1. Emergency admission
2. All age groups, but especially elderly individuals recently bereaved, socially isolated, or with sensory or mental impairment
3. Malignancy, especially cancer of the gastrointestinal tract
4. Alimentary tract diseases
5. Dysphagia or anorexia

From Dickerson (1995).

malnutrition (PEM). Dickerson (1995) identified a range of patients vulnerable to hospital-induced PEM (Table 1.2).

Malnutrition in hospital may be more common than generally thought, although the problem was recognized in 1977 (Hill *et al.* 1977). Hill's original work focused on the poor nutritional status of surgical inpatients. Approximately 30% of this group were malnourished. More recent research demonstrates that malnutrition still exists. McWhirter and Pennington found that 200 out of 500 patients admitted were undernourished, and just over 100 lost weight during their admission (McWhirter and Pennington 1994). Malnutrition can affect wound healing in several ways:

i) Poor wound healing, reduced tensile strength and increased wound dehiscence (Stotts and Whitney 1990, Dickerson 1995)
ii) Increased susceptibility to infections (Dickerson 1995)
iii) Susceptibility to the development of pressure sores (Pinchcofsky-Devin and Kaminski 1986, Hanan and Scheele 1991, Dickerson 1995)
iv) Poor-quality scarring (Pinchcofsky-Devin 1994)

Recommended daily intakes are given in Table 1.3.

Vitamin deficiency
Vitamin C is essential for the synthesis of collagen. It functions as a cofactor in the hydroxylation of proline to hydroxyproline (Pinchcofsky-Devin 1994). A deficiency in vitamin C reduces tensile strength within wounds and impairs angiogenesis and increases capillary fragility (McLaren 1992).

Table 1.3 *Recommended daily intake of energy, protein and carbohydrate*

	Energy (kcal)	Energy (kJ)	Protein (g)	Carbohydrate
Men	2150–2510	9030–1054	54–63	40–50% of daily intake
Women	1680–2150	7055–9030	42–54	40–50% of daily intake

From Barker (1991).

Vitamin A may also be linked to limiting wound infections as it is important in the normal human defence mechanism. Supplements of vitamin A have been used to reverse the effects of corticosteroid treatments in patients, to improve wound healing (Pinchcofsky-Devin 1994).

Fluid balance

In addition to an adequate intake of food, fluids are also required. Around 2000–2500 ml of fluid are required daily for efficient metabolism.

Smoking

Smoking has an adverse effect on the general health of individuals throughout their lives. There is a high correlation between smoking, lung cancer and cardiovascular diseases. Tobacco smoke contains nicotine and carbon monoxide. There are, however, differences between cigarette smoke and pipe or cigar smoke as far as nicotine is concerned, cigarettes being more harmful to health (Siana *et al.* 1992) with more nicotine being absorbed and peripheral blood flow being depressed by at least 50% for more than an hour after smoking just one cigarette. In animal models nicotine has been shown to inhibit epithelialization (Mosely *et al.* 1978); human smokers have been shown to have post-operative problems with scarring (Siana *et al.* 1989). On the other hand, no specific research has evaluated the influence of carbon monoxide on healing (Siana *et al.* 1992). There is a plethora of research on the detrimental effects of carbon monoxide on blood vessels and blood components suggestive of a probable effect on wound healing (Table 1.4).

Drug therapies

Drugs that interfere with cell proliferation have a severe effect on wound healing. These are predominantly cytotoxic drugs, especially vincristine. However, the most commonly encountered drugs that adversely affect

Table 1.4 *The main influence of nicotine and carbon monoxide on peripheral tissue in relation to wound healing*

Tissue	Nicotine	Carbon monoxide	Total effect
Skin Muscles	Contraction Dilation	Dilation Dilation	Contraction
Oxygen supply	Reduced blood flow	Reduced oxygen transport	Reduced oxygen tension in tissue
Platelets	Increased aggregation	Increased aggregation	Formation of thrombi
Fibrin	Increased plasma concentration	No proven effect	

From Siana *et al.* (1992)

healing are the corticosteroids. When taken over a long period, they suppress fibroblast and collagen synthesis.

Radiotherapy

Depending on the dosage of radiotherapy used, wounds in the immediate vicinity of the treated area may fail to heal or heal slowly. Long-term weakness of the skin and other tissue can result following radiotherapy (Irvin 1981).

Assessment of the Wound

Accurate assessment of a wound depends on the ability of the nurse to recognize both normal and abnormal healing. A sound knowledge of what is happening throughout the healing phase is the basis of accurate assessment.

Sutured Wounds

In many surgical procedures the surgeon can bring the edges of the wound together by using sutures (primary closure). Suitable procedures are:

  i) Clean surgical procedures
 ii) Procedures that result in little loss of tissue
iii) Procedures where tissues can be brought together without causing tension.

The length of time a sutured wound will take to heal depends not only on the general health of the individual, but also on the site of the incision. Where the sutured area has a good blood supply (e.g. wounds on the head and neck) healing may be completed within 3 days. Other sites may take up to 14 days. Sutures should be removed as soon as possible following healing to minimize scarring, but must be left in for long enough so that the wound does not dehisce.

A variety of suture materials are available (Table 1.5). More important than

Table 1.5 *Suture materials*

Suture materials	Strength	Tissue reaction
Absorbable:		
Dexon, Vicryl, PDS	+++	+
catgut	+	+++
Non-absorbable:		
silk, cotton	+	+++
Goretex, Ethilon, Tricron, Prolene	++	+
paper	+	+
steel	+++	++

+, weakest; +++, strongest.
PDS, polydioxanone sutures.

the choice of suture material, however, is the techique used for suturing. Surgeons are taught to follow these principles:

■ Choose the right suture for the site of the incision, the tensile strength required and the resultant scarring.

■ Use an adequate 'bite' when bringing the skin edges together. Larger 'bites' of tissue within the suture will generally result in a stronger wound.

■ Choose the appropriate method of suturing. The choice includes:
   interrupted
   interrupted — mattress
   continuous — subcuticular
   continuous — blanket
   continuous — over-and-over

■ Maintain the correct distance evenly between individual sutures.

■ Ensure adequate and even tension while suturing — too slack and the wound will not be held together in close approximation, too tight and tissue death may occur.

Note — it is possible for some wounds to be brought together and closed using paper tapes (e.g. Steri-strips or a semiocclusive dressing such as Opsite) as an alternative method.

Dressings

A great deal of debate has ensued about whether sutured wounds need to be dressed. It is usual for a simple dressing to be applied in theatre (e.g. an absorbent island dressing). This theatre dressing can safely be removed about 24–48 hours post-operatively. It is not necessary for a further dressing to be used (Chrintz *et al.* 1989). As an alternative, where little oozing is expected post-operatively, a semipermeable film (e.g. Opsite, Tegaderm) may be applied directly to the wound in theatre and left in place until the sutures need to be removed. This method had several advantages: the wound and the surrounding area may be observed easily without having to disturb dressings, and the patient can bathe.

Post-operative observations

The wound and the surrounding area should be observed at least once every 24 hours and whenever the patient complains of pain or discomfort.

In a normal, healthy, sutured wound, some degree of inflammation, swelling and redness is to be expected around 2–3 days post-operatively. This demonstrates that the wound is in the inflammatory phase of healing. However, observation should be maintained for the clinical signs of infection, which are:

■ Generalized malaise and patient complaints of feeling unwell
■ Pyrexia and tachycardia

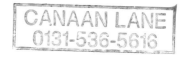

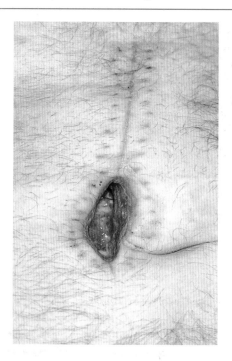

Figure 1.11 *Partial wound breakdown following cholecystectomy.*

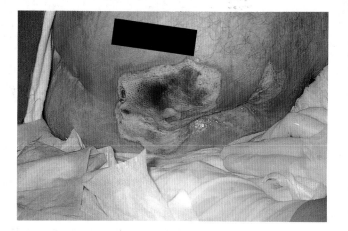

Figure 1.12 *Excessive exudate being produced by a large sacral pressure sore. Note the maceration of the skin surrounding the wound.*

- Wound beginning to discharge
- The area surrounding the wound becoming red, sore, swollen and indurated
- On removal of a suture pus is discharged
- Partial wound breakdown following removal of sutures (Figure 1.11)

Granulating Wounds

Exudate production

The amound of exudate an open wound produces can vary tremendously throughout the healing phase (Figure 1.12). In the immediate post-operative period, surgically created cavities can produce large amounts of wound exudate. It also follows that, generally, the larger the wound the more fluid it is likely to produce. It is usual for exudate production to diminish throughout the healing phase as a wound becomes smaller. Wounds, however, will continue to ooze small amounts of exudate until complete re-epithelialization has occurred.

On the other hand, wound beds which are dry are not considered to be healthy, and will need careful assessment and documentation in preparation for intervention (Figure 1.13).

Figure 1.13 *A dry wound bed on an abdominal wall wound.*

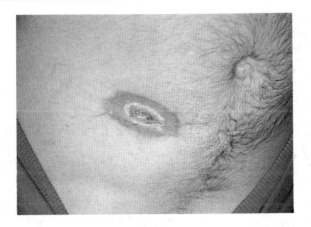

Appearance of the wound bed

The appearance of the wound bed indicates both the stage of healing and the health of the wound.

A newly created surgical cavity often appears red and raw, and has adipose tissue or muscle at the base of the wound. This appearance is normal during the first 2 weeks of healing, prior to granulation tissue being formed (Figure 1.14).

Healthy granulation tissue appears at around 14 days, and persists throughout the healing phase. It is pale pink or yellow and has a bumpy or 'cobblestone' appearance. Healthy granulation tissue is firm to touch, painless and does not bleed.

Towards the end of healing, new epithelium covers the surface of the wound. It is pale pink in colour and is usually seen at the edges of the wound, gradually creeping toward the middle to cover the wound completely (Figure 1.15).

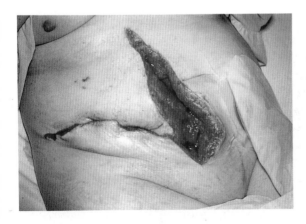

Figure 1.14 *Pregranulation. An abdominal wound three days after surgery.*

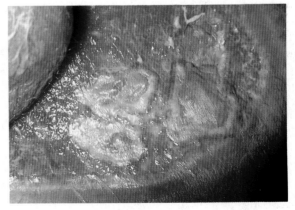

Figure 1.15 *Epithelialization.*

Slough
a mass of dead tissue in or
cast out of living tissue

Slough

Slough is most commonly seen lining the base of chronic wounds such as leg ulcers and pressure sores (Figure 1.16). It is yellow or white in appearance and consists of dead, devitalized tissue. Slough can be dry or moist and is characterized by being firmly adherent to the base of the wound.

Necrotic tissue

Necrotic tissue is often seen in conjunction with slough. Necrotic tissue is black or blackish green in appearance and, like slough, consists of dead tissue, commonly associated with chronic wounds (Figure 1.17). Necrotic tissue can be hard and leathery in appearance, or soft and moist. As with slough, it is firmly stuck to the wound bed.

Hypergranulation
exhuberant amounts of soft,
oedematous granulation
tissue developing during
healing

Hypergranulation

Occasionally re-epithelialization fails to take place owing to the presence of excessive granulation tissue (**hypergranulation** or proud flesh). Epithelial

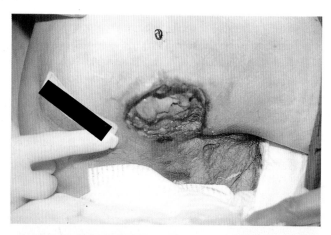

Figure 1.16 *Sloughy tissue on the wound bed of a stage IV pressure sore with underlying extensive tissue damage.*

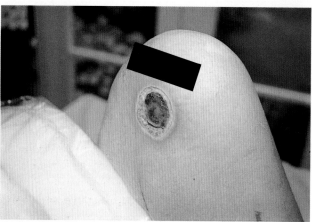

Figure 1.17 *Necrotic tissue covering a pressure sore on the inner aspect of the knee.*

migration cannot continue over hypergranulation, and this tissue needs to be flattened to effect complete healing through re-epithelialization.

Wound Shape

It is important to recognize the importance of wound shape and its effect on healing. Ideally, surgically created cavities should be boat-shaped or saucer-shaped, with evenly sloping sides. This allows free drainage of wound secretions and enables easy dressing of the wound. Many chronic wounds, especially pressure sores, are irregularly shaped with undermining pockets, tracts and sinuses. Where these are present, drainage of wound secretions is inadequate, encouraging wound infection. Poor wound shape also restricts the range of dressing materials that can be used. Occasionally wound shape is so poor and progress towards healing is so slow that surgical revision may be needed to give the wound more regular contours.

Wound Size

Generally, the larger the wound the longer it will take to heal, so it is possible, in some wound types, to predict when wounds of a given size should heal. This is possible for pilonidal sinus excisions and abdominal wall wounds (Marks *et al.* 1983).

Wound size can be difficult to measure accurately and there are several methods of doing this. Measurement of the wound can help in the evaluation of healing (see Chapter 8).

Wound Infection

Bacteria
any prokaryotic organism

Wound infection can occur at any time during the healing phase, and all types of wound can become infected (Figures 1.18, 1.19). All wounds are colonized with **bacteria** which do not necessarily delay or affect healing; however, pathogenic organisms growing in large numbers are likely to produce wound infection. Some patients are more vulnerable to infection than others.

Pathogenic organisms that commonly cause wound infection are listed below.

Aerobic bacteria

Aerobic bacteria thrive in the presence of oxygen but do not necessarily depend upon it.

- *Staphylococcus aureus* is carried by around 30% of the population and causes many hospital-acquired wound infections.
- *Staphylococcus epidermidis* is found in large quantities on the intact skin of individuals. *Staphylococcus epidermidis* is present in the air and in dust, being constantly shed by the skin, and counts are expecially high when people are frequently moving around in enclosed spaces.
- Methicillin-resistant *Staphylococcus aureus* (MRSA) has been a cause of hospital-acquired infection for many years. With the discovery of

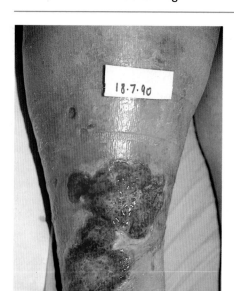

18·7·90

Figure 1.18   *An infected venous leg ulcer showing unhealthy granulation tissue and maceration of the surrounding skin.*

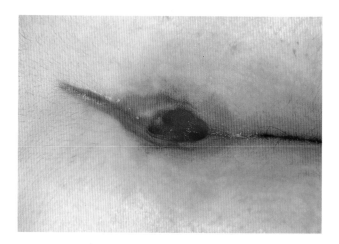

Figure 1.19   *Infection occurring during healing of a pilonidal sinus wound. Note the unhealthy appearance of the granulation tissue. An anaerobic organism has been cultured from this wound.*

penicillin serious outbreaks of hospital-acquired infections were brought under control. Unfortunately *Staphylococcus aureus* quickly developed resistance to penicillin. The emergence of MRSA was reported in 1961 (Jevans 1961) and it has been causing problems ever since (Siu 1994), especially in intensive care units and elderly care wards. Methods of spread include the unwashed hands of doctors and nurses, contact with heavily contaminated families and surfaces, and airborne spread from infected patients (Siu 1994). A high incidence of sepsis and serious complications occur in seriously ill patients, including those who have suffered burns or who are immunocompromised (Simpson 1992).

■ Beta-haemolytic streptococci are found in around 5% of the population and more commonly in those suffering from acute tonsillitis. In burns and plastic surgery units this bacteria causes infection under skin grafts and can lead to the death of the graft.

■ *Escherichia coli* and *Proteus* are normal bowel flora. These bacteria can be spread by hand contamination or by local approximation of the perineum to the wound. Sacral pressure sores are prime candidates for such contamination, especially if the patient is incontinent of faeces. Occasionally spillage may occur during intestinal surgery which contaminates the surgical incision.

- *Klebsiella* and *Pseudomonas* (Figure 1.20) are found in moist conditions although they are also normal bowel commensals. Because they are free-living these bacteria can easily contaminate lotions and antiseptics. Flower vases and water used for chrysanthemums are particular sources of *Pseudomonas*; it is also common in sinks and sluices.

Anaerobic bacteria

Anaerobic bacteria
bacteria which thrive in an
anoxic environment

Anaerobic bacteria thrive in the absence of oxygen and so are suited to the conditions found in the bowel and in soil.

- *Bacteroides* is present in large numbers in the bowels of healthy individuals. In pilonidal sinus excisions these micro-organisms are responsible for an infection rate of around 20%, owing to the close proximity of these wounds to the anus. Leakage during bowel surgery can cause peritonitis.
- *Clostridium welchii* is a potentially fatal organism. This spore-bearing organism is present in the bowel and in soil and when it contaminates a wound it can cause gas gangrene. Poorly perfused wound sites such as amputation stumps or deep contaminated traumatic cavities are especially at risk.
- *Clostridium tetani* is another spore-bearing organism which infects wounds that have been exposed to dirt or soil where these bacteria are commonly found, causing tetanus in the unprotected individual.

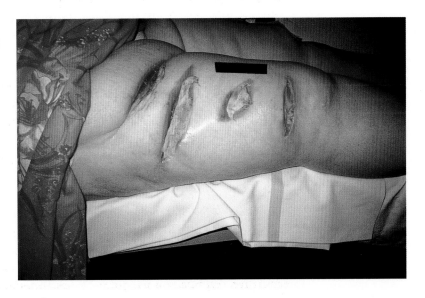

Figure 1.20 *Abscess excision sites infected with* Pseudomonas. *Note the blue-green discharge characteristic of* Pseudomonas.

Figure 1.21   *Sources of infection in hospital.*

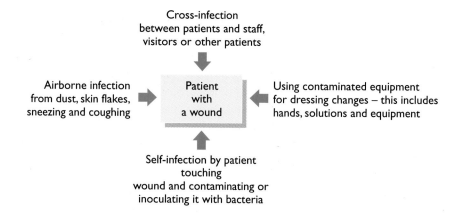

Susceptible patients

Patients who are susceptible to developing wound infection include:

i) The immunocompromised or patients with a debilitating illness

Devitalized
devoid of vitality or life; dead

ii) Patients with **devitalized** tissue in their wound

iii) Patients with a haematoma in their wound

iv) Patients with a poor blood supply to the wound

v) Patients who are at risk of contamination of their wound, e.g. through dementia or incontinence

vi) Older patients — advancing age increases the risk of wound infection (Mishriki *et al.* 1990)

vii) Obese patients — gross obesity increases the risk of wound infection (Cruse and Foord 1973)

viii) Patients who are shaved pre-operatively or who stay in hospital for longer than 7 days pre-operatively (Cruse and Foord 1980)

Possible routes of infection in patients with wounds are shown in Figure 1.21.

Possible causes of wound infection

Wound infection does not occur in all situations where pathogenic organisms are found, but depends on the number of pathogens, their virulence and the host's resistance to infection. The following formula is the recognized method of calculating the likelihood of infection developing (Westaby and White 1985):

$$\frac{\text{number of organisms} \times \text{virulence}}{\text{host's resistance}}$$

Clinical signs of infection

Infected granulation tissue (Figure 1.22) has an appearance characterized by:

- Flimsy, friable granulation tissue
- Superficial bridging within the wound
- Spontaneous bleeding or bleeding on light contact
- Pain or discomfort within the wound
- Delayed healing or wound enlargement
- Offensive wound exudate
- Pus secretion
- **Cellulitis** or inflammation in the tissues surrounding the wound

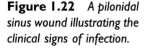
Cellulitis
inflammation of the
subcutaneous tissues

Infection in primary wound closure is characterized by:

- Redness, inflammation and induration of the tissues surrounding the wound (not associated with the immediate post-operative inflammatory phase of healing, which is a normal phenomenon occurring around days 1–3 following surgery)
- Partial wound breakdown accompanied by a discharge of pus or haemo-serous fluid
- Pain, throbbing and heat in the wound area and surrounding tissues

It is usually necessary to take a sample of wound exudate or discharge for culture and sensitivity by the bacteriology laboratory. Identifying the organism causing the wound infection, together with its sensitivity to an antibiotic, facilitates early treatment of the wound infection. Wound swabs are best taken using an aseptic technique, gathering as much exudate as possible without contaminating the sterile swab with skin flora. The swab should be sent to the laboratory as soon as possible, within 24 hours at the latest, using a transport medium where appropriate.

Assessment of the Environment

The final step in this organized approach considers the physical and social environment in which the individual is being cared for. Having a wound is likely to have a profound effect on the individual's lifestyle.

Figure 1.22 *A pilonidal sinus wound illustrating the clinical signs of infection.*

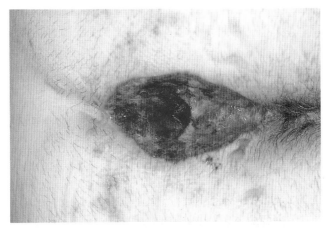

Hospital-based Care

Consideration should be given to the type of area the patient is being nursed in, for example the accident and emergency, care of the elderly, paediatric or psychiatric department.

Community-based Care

Care may be provided in the patient's own home, nursing home, residential home, school or college, or work-place. The providers of care and support should be assessed, as well as the physical cleanliness of the environment. The effects of social class on expectations and knowledge can also determine the management of the patient. As with David Simons in Case Study 1.1, care may be given in a range of environments, spanning hospital, hospice and then council housing. Mr Simons' wife was unwilling and unable to provide care when he finally went home, thus support was required from the community services.

Summary

This chapter has covered all aspects that need to be considered when assessing any patient with a wound, whether simple or complex. Before proceeding to the next chapter reflect on these aspects, which are:

■ Assessment of the individual:
  recognizing the stages of normal healing
  recognizing abnormal healing processes
  wound healing by primary or secondary intention

■ Factors that affect healing:
  intrinsic
  extrinsic

■ Assessment of the wound:
  sutured or granulating
  shape and size
  infection

■ Assessment of the environment:
  hospital-based
  community-based
  caregivers

The way in which all these aspects can be used in an organized framework is discussed in the next chapter.

Further Reading

Bucknall TE & Ellis H (eds) (1984) *Wound Healing for Surgeons*. London: Baillière Tindall.

Weiss JB and Aynd S (1982) An introduction to collagen. In Weiss JS & Joyson MIV (eds) *Collagen in Health and Disease*. Edinburgh: Churchill Livingstone.

Cohen IK & McCoy BJ (1980) The biology and control of surface over-healing. *World Journal of Surgery* 4: 298–295.

Cohen IK, Dieglemann RF & Lindbland WJ (1992) *Wound Healing: Biochemical and Clinical Aspects*. London: WB Saunders.

Adzick NS & Longaker MT (eds) (1991) *Total Wound Healing*. New York: Elsevier.

Butterworth RJ (1993) Wound contraction: a review. *Journal of Wound Care* 2(3): 172–175.

Lawrence JC, Nelson EA & Turner TD (1995) Review of classic research: moist wound healing. *Journal of Wound Care* 4(8): 366–371.

Barker HM (1991). *Beck's Nutrition and Dietetics for Nurses*. Edinburgh: Churchill Livingstone.

References

Adam K & Oswald I (1983) Protein synthesis, body renewal and the sleep-wake cycle. *Science* 165: 513–515.

Barker HM (1991) *Beck's Nutrition and Dietetics for Nurses*. Edinburgh: Churchill Livingstone.

Centre for Medical Education (1992) *The Wound Programme*. University of Dundee.

Chrintz H, Vibits H, Cordtz TO *et al* (1989) Need for surgical wound dressing. *British Journal of Surgery* 76: 204–205.

Cruse PJE & Foord R (1973) A five-year prospective study of 23,649 surgical wounds. *Archives of Surgery* 107: 206–217.

Cruse PJE & Foord R (1980) The epidemiology of wound infection: a 10 year prospective study of 62,939 wounds. *Surgical Clinics of North America* 60(12): 27–40.

Dealey C (1994) The management of patients with wounds. In: *The Care of Wounds*. Oxford: Blackwell.

Deitch EA & Bridges RM (1987) Stress hormones modulate neutrophil and lymphocyte activity *in vitro*. *Journal of Trauma* 27(10): 1146–1154.

Dickerson J (1995) The problem of hospital induced malnutrition. *Nursing Times* Jan 25, 92(4): 44–45.

Hanan K & Scheele L (1991) Albumin vs weight as a predictor of nutritional status and pressure ulcer development. *Ostomy Wound Management* 33: 2, 22–27.

Heiss J (1976) *Family Roles and Intervention*, 2nd edn. Chicago: Rand McNally.

Hill GL, Pickford I, Young GA *et al* (1977) Malnutrition in surgical patients: an unrecognised problem. *Lancet* i: 689–692.

Irvin, TT (1981) *Wound Healing: Principles and Practice*. London: Chapman & Hall.

Jevans MP (1961) 'Celbenci'-resistant staphylococcus. *British Medical Journal* 1: 124.

Maier SF & Laudenslager M (1985) Stress and health: exploring the links. *Psychology Today* 19(8): 44–49.

Marks J, Hughes LE, Harding KG, Campbell H, Ribeiro CD (1983). Prediction of healing time as an aid to the management of open granulating wounds. *World Journal of Surgery*, 7: 41–45.

McLaren SMG (1992) Nutrition and wound healing. *Journal of Wound Care* 1(3): 45–55.

McWhirter JP & Pennington C (1994) Incidence and recognition of malnutrition in hospital. *British Medical Journal* 308: 945–948.

Mishriki SF, Law DJW & Jeffrey PJ (1990) Factors affecting the incidence of post operative wound infection. *Journal of Hospital Infection* 16: 223–230.

Mosely LM, Finsett F & Goody M (1978) Nicotine and its effect on wound healing. *Plastic and Reconstructive Surgery* 61: 570–575.

Pinchcofsky-Devin G (1994) Nutritional wound healing. *Journal of Wound Care* 3(5): 231–234.

Pinchcofsky-Devin GD & Kaminski MV (1986) Correlation of pressure sores and nutritional status. *Journal of the American Geriatrics Society* 34: 435–440.

Rigby H (1992) Tissue healing, Part 1. *Surgery* 10(11): 261–264.

Siana JE, Rex S & Gottrup F (1989) The effect of cigarette smoking on wound healing. *Scandinavian Journal of Plastic and Reconstructive Surgery*, 23: 207–209.

Siana, JE, Frankild BS & Gottrup F (1992) The effect of smoking on tissue function. *Journal of Wound Care* July/Aug, 1(2): 37–41.

Silver, IA (1994) The physiology of wound healing. *Journal of Wound Care* 3(2): 106–109.

Simpson S (1992) Methicillin-resistant *Staphylococcus aureus* and its implications for nursing practice: literature review. *Nursing Practice* 5(2): 2–7.

Siu ACK (1994). Methicillin-resistant *Staphylococcus aureus*: do we just have to live with it? *British Journal of Nursing* 3(15): 753–759.

Stotts NA & Whitney JD (1990) Nutritional intake and status of clients in the home with open surgical wounds. *Journal of Community Nursing* 7(2): 77–86.

Westaby S & White S (1985) Wound infection. In Westaby S (ed) *Wound Care*. London: William Heinemann Medical Books Ltd.

Whitby DJ (1995) The biology of wound healing. *Surgery* 13(2): 25–28.

2 Assessing and Planning Individualized Care

Key issues

This chapter gives an overview of nursing theory and the basis of nursing models which are used as a framework for assessing patients with wounds. Nursing models are classified and outlined as follows:

Developmental

- Peplau's model
- Orem's model

Systems

- Roy's model
- Roper, Logan and Tierney's model

Interaction

- Riehl's model
- Goal setting and outcomes are also covered.

Introduction

Assessing a patient with a wound can prove to be difficult, especially for the inexperienced practitioner.

There are many ways in which nurses assess their patients: some haphazardly, some using a medical model framework, and others using a nursing model. In order to use a nursing model, nurses must understand the basis of the model. In the right circumstances nursing models can provide a clear framework for practitioners to follow as well as providing an optimum level of care for the patient.

This chapter explains the theory that underpins nursing models and explains the type of patient they might be best suited for.

It is important when using an organized framework to identify patient problems, that clear goals and outcomes are identified. The setting of goals and outcomes is explained using examples of particular wound types.

Using a Nursing Model to Assess Individuals

Before a nursing model is used it is important that the nurse understands the basis of the nursing theory that underpins it. Often this vital step is overlooked, as models are frequently introduced via the curriculum of a college of nursing or on a regional basis throughout all the clinical areas within a health authority. This only adds to the resistance to using a model, as nurses fail to understand the philosophy behind the model or its relevance to practice.

Theoretical Basis of Models

It is difficult in the early stages of a nursing career to understand what 'nursing' is all about. The use of models may be one way in which nursing and nursing care can be examined. Wright (1986) sees models as a continuing process of critical thinking about nursing.

It is in this way that nursing theory can be developed alongside the model, but not in isolation from practice. One of the major complaints from practitioners is that often nursing theory has little or no relevance to clinical practice. Because models are often imposed or dictated, nurses do not have the flexibility to discover how, or which, model fits into their line of practice. Models must be suited to the patients' needs, not vice versa.

Of equal importance is the relationship between the use of models and the nursing process. The nursing process, a system of individualized nursing care, is achieved with the use of a nursing model — it is not a nursing model itself, and this distinction must be made clear. So, how can the application of a nursing model help to decrease the gap between theory and practice?

Wound management is so obviously a practical subject that it can be used as a focus for the use of a model while drawing continually on the biological and behavioural scientific knowledge that underpins its practice (Figure 2.1). Using a model as a framework can help students and inexperienced practitioners bring structure into what may appear a myriad of theories, abstract concepts, haphazard treatment and intuitive behaviour. However, models are constructed on the assumption that patient-centred care is in use (Kershaw and Salvage 1986), and often on busy wards with staff shortages task allocation may be in use under the pretence that a model of nursing is practised. This is confusing to students who may construe this situation as the model not working, hence contributing to the 'theory–practice gap' (Cook 1991). In certain circumstances the model may need to be set aside in

Figure 2.1 *Wound management theory. (Adapted from Akinsanya 1984.)*

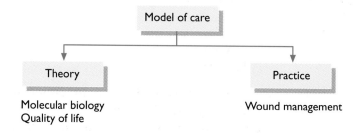

place of a system that prioritizes patients' needs, which are assessed and planned on a less formal basis. This informal method of care is often practised by 'experienced' nurses who feel they do not need a designated model, but set their own framework through which they practise. This informal, unsystematic way of working is very difficult to pass on to others as it is often based on intuitive and ritualistic care that has little theoretical foundation (Walsh and Ford 1989).

Theories and models of nursing address four concepts:

- The individual
- Society or the environment of care
- Health
- Nursing, its nature and role (Perry and Jolley 1991)

Deductive or inductive approach

Models are based on either a deductive or an inductive approach. These terms are derived from the physical sciences, as is the concept of using models, which originally were physical representations of physical objects. Later on, the behavioural sciences adopted the use of models to predict behaviour.

The laws of physical science were established through the formulation of hypotheses which were then formally tested by experimental methods. This is known as the deductive method; it relies heavily on controlling the variables under study, and is not always suitable for the behavioural sciences such as psychology and sociology. During the 1960s sociologists found that the generation of theory was better achieved by observation of practice and behaviour. This is the inductive approach to theory generation, and has been found to be very suitable to nursing studies. It also facilitated the move away from the medical model of care, as medical knowledge is largely based on the deductive method of theory generation. This shift has not been an easy or comfortable move for many nurses, and often nursing models are still used as medical models. This is highlighted in Table 2.1, which is an example of the Roper activities of living model (Roper *et al.* 1983) in use on a medical ward. The problems identified are largely medical conditions and symptoms, such as renal failure and dehydration, and it is this framework that is used by the ward nurses.

Classification of Models

Models can be classified according to their underpinning theory, as follows:

- Developmental
- Systems
- Interaction

However, many models will not be totally illuminated by one underlying philosophy but will contain aspects of two or even all three theories. This can often lead to confusion when trying to establish the theoretical

Table 2.1 *A patient's problems. Activities of living have been grouped according to their degree of correspondence to physiological systems. (P) indicates a potential problem*

Activity of living	Problem statements
Maintaining a safe environment	Risk of self-injury (P)
Communicating	Diminished verbal response Anxiety, depression Accent
Breathing	Cough Infected sputum Pain Dyspnoea Cigarette smoking
Eating and drinking	Anorexia Dehydration Poor dentition Oral infection (P)
Elimination	Renal failure (P) Renal infection (P) Constipation (P)
Personal cleansing and dressing	Inability or unwillingness to care for self Excessive perspiration
Controlling body temperature	Dehydration (P)
Mobilizing	Immobility Pressure sores (P) Deep vein thrombosis Exacerbation of chest infection
Working and playing	
Expressing sexuality	
Sleeping	
Dying	Non-acceptance of nature of disease (P)

From Roper *et al* (1983).

underpinnings of a particular model. The models used in this book are categorized according to their *primary* focus.

Developmental models

Developmental models focus on theories of development or change (Kershaw and Salvage 1986). These theories centre around how a person is developing and how nursing can help when normal development is threatened or impaired.

In the developmental process stages follow a predictable course and proceed in an orderly fashion, even towards illness or death (Pearson and

Vaughan 1986). Development covers not just the physical, but psychological and social processes as well (Walsh 1991). Developmental models focus on helping the patient attain new developmental goals or re-establishing a developmental stage from which the patient has regressed. The two best-known models in this category are those of Peplau (1952) and Orem (1980).

Peplau's model

Hildegard Peplau was one of the first American theorists to address the changing needs of nursing (Peplau 1952). She recognized that often the care that a patient *needs* may well be different from what the patient *wants*.

Believing that nursing was based on the formation of a relationship between nurse and client, she stressed the importance of the roles and phases through which nurse and patient pass during the interpersonal process. The first purpose of the nurse is to ensure survival of the patients, the second is to help them understand and come to terms with their health problems. For example, when a patient with diabetes mellitus has a foot amputated because of ischaemia, the first concern of the nurse is control of the diabetes and infection. Both conditions, unchecked, are life-threatening. The nurse's second concern is to help the patient come to terms with the loss of a foot and learn how to mobilize again.

In moving towards health the patient moves through four phases: orientation, identification, exploration and resolution. These four phases correspond to the four phases of the nursing process.

- Orientation (assessment):
    nurse learns the nature of the difficulty the patient is experiencing
    development of mutual trust
    problem identification
- Identification (planning):
    recognition by the patient of the formulation of the nurse–patient relationship
    nurse plans appropriate intervention
- Exploitation (implementation):
    patient recognizes and responds to services offered by the nurse
    interpersonal relationship is fully established
    both nurse and patient move towards mutual goals
- Resolution (evaluation):
    health problem resolved or improved
    nursing input no longer required, or at minimal level
    patient returns to independence
    new goals or existing developmental stage re-established

Peplau's model has no particular framework or form of record-keeping to be used during the assessment phase. She advocates the use of the acronym SOAP:

S — the *subjective experience* as described by the patient
O — *objective observation* made by the nurse
A — *formal assessment* and identification of problems (based on S and O)
P — *plan* of action

For an example, look at Case Study 4.3.

Orem's self-care model
Orem's framework has been classified as a systems model (Riehl and Roy 1980) or simply as a self-care model (Aggleton and Chalmers 1986; Pearson and Vaughan 1986). However, Fawcett (1989) and Walsh (1991) agreed that Orem's model demonstrates strong characteristics of a developmental model. The model emphasizes the concept of self-care where people take responsibility for their own healthcare, which is provided where possible by friends and family. The model rejects the passive role of the patient and is more in tune with today's nursing, which allows patients to participate in their own care.

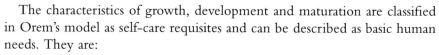

The characteristics of growth, development and maturation are classified in Orem's model as self-care requisites and can be described as basic human needs. They are:

- Sufficient intake of air
- Sufficient intake of water
- Sufficient intake of food
- Satisfactory eliminator functions
- Activity balanced with rest
- Time spent alone balanced with time spent with others
- Prevention of danger to self
- Being normal

Two further self-care requisites are described:

- *Developmental self-care requisites:* these may affect the universal self-care requisites according to the stage of development of the individual or the environment in which the individual lives.
- *Health deviation self-care requisites:* ill-health or disability may necessitate a change in self-care behaviour.

Self-care is possible when individuals are able to cope with the demands placed upon them. When these demands become too great, or the individual's ability to cope decreases, then an imbalance occurs, causing a 'self-care deficit'.

Assessment using Orem's model should be carried out in two stages:

Stage 1 — Establishing *if there is* a self-care deficit.
Stage 2 — If there is, *why there is* a self-care deficit — is it because the patient

lacks knowledge, skill or motivation, or has a limited range of behaviour?

Having identified a self-care deficit, the nurse should plan — with the patient where possible — the goals of care.

The nurse must decide whether the intervention will be:

i)   Wholly compensatory, i.e. the nurse acts for the patient completely
ii) Partly compensatory, i.e. certain aspects of care are shared by patient and nurse
iii) Educative–developmental, i.e. the nurse gives the patient the necessary knowledge or skills to allow self-care

The level at which the patient is involved in planning care will depend on the patient's physical and mental state, but the nurse should always aim to maximize the patient's input where possible. The patient's relatives or carers should be included in this planning as they may be a key factor in helping the patient achieve this potential.

Nursing *intervention* follows the planning stage. Orem has distinguished five methods of implementing the care plan:

i)   acting or doing for another
ii) guiding another
iii) supporting another, physically or psychologically
iv) providing an environment that promotes personal development
v)   teaching another

The move from dependency to independence is clear in this model. It must be stressed, however, that giving a patient a task to do without assessing the patient's potential is not self-care and may have dire consequences, as in Case Study 2.1. With proper assessment and planning this situation could have been avoided. Can you see why it occurred?

Case Study 2.1   Mr Steven Jones is a 22-year-old student who has undergone surgery for an excision of pilonidal sinus. He is anxious to return home and to his studies as he has examinations in 6 weeks' time.

The nurse explains verbally how he can change his foam dressing himself. She does not:
i)   enquire if he has a carer (partner or parent) who could assist the dressing change
ii) explain the importance of cleansing his foam 'bung' twice daily
iii) watch Steven doing the dressing change before discharge
iv) explain the importance of personal hygiene
v)   give any written explanation

Steven goes home with his dressings, but without support at home and without any kind of written guidance, he quickly forgets what he has to do. He consequently rings his general practitioner who sends the district nurse to the house to help with the dressing change. The district nurse is annoyed with Steven and the hospital as she feels this to be an unnecessary call, when she has many less able patients to call on. Steven feels stupid and inadequate that he is unable to cope.

Systems models

Systems models are characterized by the progression along a life-span, the examination of the system, its parts and their relationship with each other at a given time.

The major features of systems models are the system and its environment. It is how the system reacts to the environment and maintains its equilibrium that is of major interest. In contrast to developmental models, change is of secondary importance. Systems models are concerned with maintaining a balance along the life-span; although each part is studied separately, interaction of the parts is most important (Pearson and Vaughan 1986).

'System' and 'environment' are defined according to the context of study, e.g. a system could be a person whose parts are body organs and whose environment is the family.

Systems may be open or closed. An open system is one of continuous inflow and outflow, the outflow becoming the inflow for the next stage of the system, and so on. Open systems are therefore influenced by internal and external factors; the less interference from either of these factors, the more smoothly the system will run.

As in the human body, a disturbance within the function of one of the internal subsystems or external factors will produce an imbalance. In order for the body to maintain homeostasis a new balance has to be achieved. This may be self-regulated, for example the production of insulin for the conversion of glucose to give energy. Outside intervention from medical and nursing staff will be required when the body is unable to regulate an imbalance; for example, when a patient has a wound infection the initial reaction by the body will be an increase in the number of white blood cells (i.e. a lymphatic response) and also a cardiovascular response, producing the signs and symptoms of infection. With the output the patient experiences pain, which subsequently becomes an input (Figure 2.2).

Understanding this systems approach will help the nurse to identify priorities of care and provide intervention that will minimize further complications or deterioration. This method of care is proactive rather than reactive, i.e. it deals with a problem before it arises rather than after.

Two models that have a distinct systems approach are Roy's adaptation

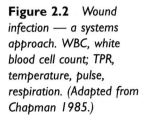

Figure 2.2 *Wound infection — a systems approach. WBC, white blood cell count; TPR, temperature, pulse, respiration. (Adapted from Chapman 1985.)*

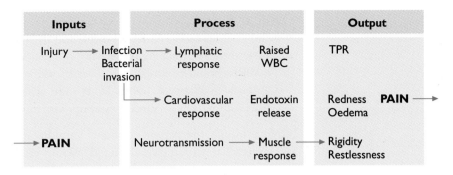

model (Roy 1980) and Roper, Logan and Tierney's activities of living model (Roper *et al.* 1980).

Roy's adaptation model
Calista Roy began developing this model in the mid-1960s in California. She sees the person as an individual whose behaviour is governed by a set of interrelated biological, psychological and social systems (Aggleton and Chalmers 1986). In order to maintain a balance individuals are in a constant state of interaction, both within themselves and with their relationship with the outside world (Roy 1971). Demands or stressors can be anything experienced in life, and how an individual copes or adapts to these will vary from person to person. It is the nurse's ability to identify stressors that will influence the patient's recovery. When the nurse is able to do this his/her role should be to promote the patient's ability to adapt and cope with the new demands. However, a person's response to stressors can vary. Roy argues that this is controlled by three sets of stimuli:

- Focal — those immediately present for the individual
- Contextual — those occurring alongside the focal stimuli
- Residual — those occurring from past learning and its effects

As these three types of stimuli will never occur in exactly the same way at any one time, the response or adaptation will also vary. Consider the example of a patient who attends an outpatient clinic on two occasions for a wound dressing:

- Visit 1:
    the clinic is busy, many patients are waiting and the room is hot (contextual stimuli)
    the nurse attending him has had no lunch break, forgets his name and cannot remember what type of operation he has had (focal stimuli)
    on his last visit the wound was infected and the doctor applied a silver nitrate stick to some overgranulation; this was extremely painful (residual stimuli)
    how do you think the patient coped with this visit?

- Visit 2:

    the clinic is quiet, cool and calm, and the patient is asked to go straight in without waiting (contextual)

    a different nurse attends this week, who addresses him by his name, appears to know all about his wound and operation and explains the procedures. The wound is healthy with no complications (focal)

Now, although the patient's residual stimulus remains the same, both focal and contextual stimuli have changed. Would you expect the same behaviour on this visit?

Roy identified four principal adaptation systems that influence behaviour:

- *Physiological system* — the body's responses to food, fluids, oxygen, circulation, temperature, sensory input, exercise and rest.

- *Self-concept system* — the view that people hold of themselves, both physically and psychologically. It is concerned with how people see their own worth, both in their own eyes and in those of others.

- *Role mastery system* — focuses on the individual's need to have a place in society: the duties and responsibilities or rights and privileges they hold.

- *Interdependency system* — the balance between dependence and independence in relationships with others. Levels of friendliness, dominance and competitiveness.

Nursing intervention will be required when there is a deficit or excess within one or more of these adaptation systems.

Assessment using Roy's model, as with other nursing models, consists of two stages. In the first stage the nurse will observe behaviour using each of the four adaptation systems as a framework. If there appears to be a problem of adaptation the nurse should move on to identify whether the factors creating this problem are focal, contextual or residual.

Planning must then identify the patient-centred goals in order of priority and the type of nursing intervention required to change either the stimuli or the patient adaptation level.

Nursing will generally concentrate on the focal stimuli as these will possibly be the primary cause of the patient's behaviour. However, this model is well suited to nurses experienced in behaviour modification and counselling techniques who have the confidence and capability to change adaptive behaviour caused by residual stimuli.

Roy's model has also been used as the model of choice for patients nursed in a terminal care setting, where the patient's and family's response to illness is essential for a balanced view, especially in changes of body image (Chadderton 1986).

Table 2.2   Activities of living

1.	Maintaining a safe environment
2.	Communicating
3.	Breathing
4.	Eating and drinking
5.	Eliminating
6.	Personal cleansing and dressing
7.	Controlling body temperature
8.	Mobilizing
9.	Working and playing
10.	Expressing sexuality
11.	Sleeping
12.	Dying

From Roper *et al.* (1980).

Roper's activities of living model

Nancy Roper's original model was the work of a research project undertaken between 1970 and 1974, and was a modification of the previous work on Virginia Henderson's model published in 1966 (Roper *et al.* 1980). It was the first attempt by British nurses at using a conceptual model to form a basis of care. The focus of the model is on twelve activities of living (Table 2.2); it acknowledges that all individuals are involved in activities that enable them to live and grow (Pearson and Vaughan 1986). The model embraces the concept of an individual progressing along a continuum with varying degrees of dependence and independence, according to age and health. Movement can be in either direction, and it should not be assumed that everyone can reach their full potential in all twelve activities. The key to using this model is the nurse's ability to assess the person's level of independence in each of the activities of living. Patient goals should be centred around the amount of nursing help required to move along the dependence/independence continuum.

For each activity of living listed in Table 2.2, the nurse should establish:

- What the patient can normally do
- What the patient can do now
- What the patient cannot do now
- What problems may develop

The assessment should, where possible, involve both patient and nurse in the process of identifying actual and potential problems. Not all activities may be a cause of problems; the nurse should, as always, prioritize the goals of care.

Nursing intervention will follow three models of action, as identified by Roper:

i)   Prevention strategies
ii) Providing comfort (physical and mental)
iii) Enabling the patient to seek help to take responsibility for self-care

This model is widely used in nursing in the UK, and has been criticized as following the medical model on the grounds that the activities of living are equivalent to physiological responses. However, this is largely due to this model being used in an inappropriate way through misunderstanding.

Interaction models

Interaction models emphasize the social meanings people put upon all aspects of their life and the interpersonal relationships between individuals. This study of interaction between people originates from the theory of the symbolic interactionism which postulates that the importance of social life lies in providing the person with language, self-concept and role-taking ability (Heiss 1976). The major focuses of such nursing models are therefore perception, communication, role and self-concept (Fawcett 1989). The key to using this type of model is to elicit the *patient's definition* of the situation, thus the model strongly identifies the active role an individual plays in any interaction.

These models therefore are unsuited to a philosophy of care that perpetuates the notion that the patient should be passive and the nurse active. Obviously in areas such as intensive care nursing, when the patient is unconscious, the nurses' active role is necessary, but in many areas of wound care interaction with patients is a central facet of management. The most widely used model from this school of thought is the Riehl interaction model (Riehl 1980).

Riehl interaction model

Riehl pays particular attention to the importance of the psychological and sociological systems or parameters and underplays the importance of physiological systems as the primary focus of nursing problems. She believes that the essence of good assessment is when nurses attempt to 'enter the subjective world of patients'. It is only then the nurse is able to help a patient adopt a more appropriate behaviour or role.

Nursing problems arise when there are disturbances within one or more of the three parameters — psychological, sociological or physiological.

Riehl does not give a particular assessment framework, but suggests the use of the FANCAP mnemonic (Abbey 1980) — Fluids, Aeration, Nutrition, Communication, Activity, Pain. The FANCAP system was originally designed as a teaching tool, and provides a bridge between nursing science and the patient.

In the first stage of assessment the nurse ascertains if the patient is adopting a role appropriate to the present situation. If there appears to be a disturbance in role, is it due to physiological, psychological or sociological parameters?

Patient-centred goals should then be identified, and activities planned for patient and nurses.

Nursing intervention will centre on role-playing, thus extending the range of behaviour open to the patient and increasing the nurses' understanding of the patient's problem.

The interaction model offers an approach that is very different from system or developmental models. It has been used widely in psychiatric nursing, where the emphasis is on psychological and social problems. It is unlikely to find popularity in mainstream areas of wound management, but can be useful when caring for patients with factitious or self-inflicted wounds (see Chapter 6).

Planning Individualized Care

It is important when assessing the patient to consider the outcome or goal that is to be achieved. This is often the most difficult part of the problem-solving process (Sparrow and Pearson 1985), especially for the inexperienced nurse. Often goals are formulated around what the nurse is trying to achieve, and not what the patient may want.

Setting Goals and Outcomes for Patients with Wounds

It is essential that the aims of management are established following assessment, as without them care will lack direction and evaluation will be impossible. This is not to say that once goals have been set they can never be changed, as unforeseen events may necessitate their revision. For example, following an operation to remove her appendix, Miss Susan James, a 28-year-old secretary, wished to return to work within 2 weeks from the date of operation. Her plan of care stated this to be one of the goals. However, 7 days post-operatively she developed a wound infection which delayed healing and necessitated **antibiotic** therapy. Therefore, following evaluation of the case at 7 days it was necessary to formulate a new goal, taking into account the patient's general condition and that of the wound.

Antibiotic
a chemical substance that is able to kill or inhibit the growth of micro-organisms

Although goal setting should be patient-centred, it is in cases such as that of Susan that the nurse's professional knowledge is required to advise the patient on what is the most reasonable and safest goal. Susan may still wish to return to her employment within the original goal of 14 days, but she should be advised that this may cause further complications of healing and result in delaying the final outcome of care — complete wound healing.

Distinguishing Goals from Outcomes

Goals and outcomes are terms that are often used interchangeably and can be confusing to students. There is no set rule as to which should be used as the definitions are similar (Concise Oxford Dictionary 1982):

- *Goal*: object of effort or ambition
- *Outcome*: result, visible effect

Both refer to an end-point of care, both should be measurable and both should be evaluated against the level of care received.

It may be simpler to define by saying that an overall outcome can be achieved by the setting of step-by-step goals. To use the analogy of a football match, the *outcome* of the match is whether the teams win, lose or draw. This outcome is dictated by the number of *goals* scored during the match. The outcome of care can be considered to be the ultimate aim of management. Whether or not it is achieved will depend on reaching step-by-step goals of care the nurse and patient have set out for themselves.

Setting Outcomes

Difficulty may be experienced when setting an outcome of management for patients with wounds because of the complexity of the wound healing process and the different types of wounds encountered.

Acute wounds

For patients with acute wounds the outcome will normally be that of complete healing. Acute surgical wounds should heal within a predicted period without complication. Work by Marks *et al.* (1983) demonstrated that an open granulating wound (such as excision of pilonidal sinus) will generally heal within 12–16 weeks. Therefore, when setting outcomes for a patient following this type of surgery, it is possible to be objective not only about the healing potential, but also about the time in which healing should be achieved. This is a good marker for evaluation, as there should be a predictable decrease in wound size as the days to healing progress. Failure to correspond with this may indicate that all is not well with the wound healing process.

Although acute wounds may be easier to evaluate in terms of healing time, it should be remembered that healing is not always the desired outcome; the patient may have other motives, and the nurse should be aware that if a wound is not healing as predicted and there are no obvious clinical signs to account for this delay, other factors should be considered. Although difficult to prove, there is some evidence to support the theory of self-inflicted injury by some patients who have a desire or ulterior motive for prolonging the wound (Baragwanath and Harding 1994). It is important to remember that complete healing should not be achieved at all costs, as the management and intervention used to achieve this may compromise the patient's quality of life.

Quality of life usually becomes more of an issue when dealing with patients whose wounds are long-standing and chronic.

Chronic wounds

The outcome of care for patients with a chronic wound is more difficult to plan, as often healing will not be achieved for many months or years, if at all.

Chronic wounds are formed when predisposing conditions impair the tissue's ability to heal the damage (Centre for Medical Education 1992). It is not unusual for individuals to have lived with a leg ulcer for 30 years, or experienced an unhealed wound sinus for many months.

Malignant wounds will not be expected to heal and in most cases become worse, therefore the outcome of care is palliation. The prime objective is alleviation of distressing symptoms, thereby maximizing the patient's quality of life.

The principle, however, remains the same, that whatever the stated outcome it should be set against measurable and observable goals.

Setting Goals

Patient goals should be defined by precise criteria, which are:

- How well? — 'the standard or degree of accuracy at which we expect the patient to perform'
- Condition — 'the circumstances under which she/he is to do it'
- Patient response — 'What is it we want the patient to be able to do' (Sparrow and Pearson 1985)

It is not always easy to write clear criteria which are also measurable and observable. It is best to avoid using subjective terms such as 'know', 'understand' and 'learn', as these do not tell us very much about how or what the patient is able to do.

Example

Edwina Banks has a venous ulcer on her right leg. She is currently having compression bandaging but the nurses would like her to complement this therapy with leg elevation.

The *outcome* of the care is to achieve complete healing of the ulcer within 4–5 months. It is necessary to formulate some patient-centred goals to achieve this. Look at the following goal: does it satisfy the three criteria outlined above?

Goal: Edwina to elevate both legs at regular intervals during the day

This goal does not really comply with the criteria as it gives no indication of 'how well' we want Edwina to elevate her legs. The 'condition' under which she is to elevate them is not stated as she will not know how regular is regular! The only thing she knows is that it is to be achieved during the day. Only the 'patient response' is stated, which is that she is required to elevate her legs. No date is given as to when she is to achieve the goal by, therefore how will the nurses know when to evaluate if it is being achieved or not?

A more useful statement of the goal is as follows:

Goal: Edwina to elevate both legs at a height above heart level for 1 hour in the morning and 1 hour in the evening by 10 March

Practice points

How should this goal be written? Try to write it yourself before looking at the answer.

The goal now defines the patient response (elevation), the conditions (1 hour twice a day) and 'how well?' (at a height above heart level).

Although this goal states all the criteria, unless the nurse has fully explained *why* the patient must elevate her legs and the best way this can be achieved, this goal may seem rather daunting, or the patient may not realize the importance elevation plays in the healing process.

As previously stated, goals *must* be patient-centred and individualized. Edwina needs to know that she can achieve this goal by lying on a sofa with her feet on the arm of the sofa; however, she may not own a sofa, or may have a chest condition which prevents her from lying down. All these facts should have been ascertained during the assessment process so that this goal can be achieved by some other means.

It is still necessary to evaluate at the stated time whether Edwina has been able to achieve her goal. If not, then changes to her care programme may be required.

Planning and writing outcomes and goals can be time-consuming and difficult. They are also dependent on the practitioner's experience in deciding what is achievable for an individual patient.

Summary

This chapter has outlined ways of using a nursing model when assessing patients with different wound aetiologies nursed in a variety of settings. Nursing models are used throughout the following chapters, demonstrating their practical application in the clinical setting. Make sure you have an understanding of their theoretical basis before moving on to the next chapter.

Models are classified as:

- Developmental:
    Peplau's model (Peplau 1952)
    Orem's model (Orem 1980)

- Systems:
    Roy's adaptation model (Roy 1971)
    Roper, Logan and Tierney's activities of living model (Roper *et al.* 1980)

- Interaction:
    Riehl's interaction model (Riehl 1980)

Remember also when assessing patients to identify measurable goals and outcomes that will provide a basis for evaluation of the patient's care.

Further Reading

Bryant RA (ed.) (1992) *Acute and Chronic Wounds. Nursing Management.* St Louis: Mosby Yearbook.

Earnest VV (1993) *Clinical Skills in Nursing Practice*, 2nd edn. Philadelphia: JB Lippincott.

McQueston, Metzger C & Webb AA (1995) *Foundations of Nursing Theory.* Thousand Oaks: Sage.

Berner P & Wrukel J (1989) *The Primary of Caring. Stress and Coping in Health and Illness.* Menlo Park: Addison-Wesley.

Meleis AI (1991) *Theoretical Nursing. Development and Progress*, 2nd edn. Philadelphia: JB Lippincott.

Robinson K & Vaughan B (1992) *Knowledge for Nursing Practice.* Oxford: Butterworth-Heinemann.

Walsh M (1991) *Models in Clinical Nursing. The Way Forward.* London: Baillière Tindall.

References

Abbey J (1980) Fancap: what is it? In: Riehl JP & Roy C (eds) *Conceptual Models for Nursing Practice*, 2nd edn. New York: Appleton-Century-Crofts.

Aggleton P & Chalmers H (1986) *Nursing Models and the Nursing Process.* London: Macmillan.

Akinsanya JA (1984) The use of theories in nursing. *Nursing Times* 80(14): 59–60.

Baragwanath P & Harding KG (1994) The management of a patient with a factitious wound. *Journal of Wound Care* 3(6): 286–287.

Centre for Medical Education (1992) *The Wound Programme.* University of Dundee.

Chadderton H (1986) A stress adaptation model in terminal care. In: Kershaw B & Salvage J, (eds) *Models for Nursing.* Chichester: John Wiley.

Chapman C (1985) *Theory of Nursing: Practical Application.* London: Harper & Row.

Concise Oxford Dictionary (1982) Oxford University Press.

Cook S (1991) Mind the theory–practice gap in nursing education. *Journal of Advanced Nursing* 16: 1462–1469.

Fawcett J (1989) *Analysis and Evaluation of Conceptual Models of Nursing*, 2nd edn. Philadelphia: FA Davies.

Heiss J (1976) *Family Roles and Intervention*, 2nd edn. Chicago: Rand McNally.

Kershaw B & Salvage J (eds) (1986) *Models for Nursing.* Chichester: John Wiley.

Marks, J, Hughes LE, Harding KG, Campbell H & Ribeiro CD (1983) Prediction of healing time as an aid to the management of open granulating wounds. *World Journal of Surgery* 7: 641–645.

Orem D (1980) *Nursing — Concepts of Practice.* New York: McGraw-Hill.

Pearson A & Vaughan B (1986) *Nursing Models for Practice.* Oxford: Butterworth-Heinemann.

Peplau H (1952) *Interpersonal Relations in Nursing.* New York: GP Putnam.

Perry A & Jolley M (1991) *Nursing: a Knowledge for Practice.* London: Edward Arnold.

Riehl JP (1980) The Riehl interaction model. In: Riehl JP & Roy C (eds) *Conceptual Models for Nursing Practice*, 2nd edn. New York: Appleton-Century-Crofts.

Riehl JP & Roy C (eds) (1980) *Conceptual Models for Nursing Practice*, 2nd edn. New York: Appleton-Century-Crofts.

Roper N, Logan WW & Tierney AJ (1980) *The Elements of Nursing.* Edinburgh: Churchill Livingstone.

Roper N, Logan WW & Tierney AJ (1983) *Using a Model for Nursing.* Edinburgh: Churchill Livingstone.

Roy C (1971) Adaptation: a conceptual framework for nursing. *Nursing Outlook* 18(3): 42–45.

Roy C (1980) The Roy adaptation model. In: Riehl JP & Roy C (eds) *Conceptual Models for Nursing Practice*, 2nd edn. New York: Appleton-Century-Crofts.

Sparrow S & Pearson A (1985) Teach yourself goal setting. *Nursing Times* Oct 16, 34–35.

Walsh M (1991) *Models in Clinical Nursing: The Way Forward*. London: Baillière Tindall.

Walsh M & Ford P (1989) *Nursing: Rituals, Research and Rational Actions*. Oxford: Butterworth-Heinemann.

Wright SG (1986) *Building and Using a Model of Nursing*. London: Edward Arnold.

INTERVENTION

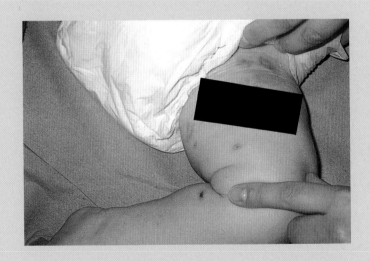

Principles of Wound Interventions

This chapter covers a whole range of interventions that will enable the reader to provide comprehensive management for patients in any range of clinical situations.
The following principles are outlined:

Development of Dressing Materials

■ Historical perspective on wound management

■ Basis of moist wound healing

■ Range of modern wound dressings

Management of Sutured and Granulating Wounds

■ Signs of infection

■ Debridement

■ Exudate production

Methods to Reduce Spread of Infection

■ Use of asceptic techniques

■ Handwashing technique

Cleansing of Wounds

■ Indications for cleansing

■ Methods of cleansing

Introduction

The sophisticated wound dressings of today are vastly superior to the small supply of gauze dressings nurses in the nineteenth century would have been able to choose from. Although dressings make a major contribution to the management of wounds, principles of cleansing, cross-infection and management of necrotic or infected tissue are also essential parts of modern wound management.

This chapter traces the history of traditional wound dressings leading up to modern dressings, basic principles and techniques which should underpin the clinical practice of all nurses involved in wound care.

Historical Perspective

The history of wound management is not only fascinating, but also helps to put today's wound management in perspective.

For early humans most wounds and injuries were the result of accidents and fighting. These injuries represented a life-threatening problem, with blood loss being a major factor; haemostasis was achieved using whatever materials came readily to hand, including sand, leaves and faeces (Knight 1985).

Cave paintings from 25 000 years ago found in Spain illustrated the common wounds found in early humans (Leaper 1986). In a history of Scandinavian folklore, Bergmark suggested that plant extracts have been used for thousands of years to treat wounds (Bergmark 1967). Some 2500 plant extracts were antimicrobial, others were astringent or were used to affect healing.

China

As surgery in China was held in low esteem, the emphasis was on prevention of illness and treatments with herbal medicines. Two famous, influential Chinese emperors, Yu Hsiung (the Yellow Emperor) and Shen Nung (the Red Emperor), compiled the first herbal treatments known as the *Pen-tsao*.

Egypt

In Egypt, surgery was rarely performed and primitive. Wound treatments included pulling the edges of wounds together with sutures made from applying sticky gum to linen strips. Primitive sutures were probably made from a thorn needle, with some type of thread (Leaper 1986). Sorcery, religion and medicine were closely related in these times. Ancient documents including a 100-page encyclopaedia of medicine found in the Ebers papyrus recorded wound healing treatments using resin, honey, lard and beef as topical agents, with stiffened bandages used for treating broken limbs. Antiseptics and astringents, in the form of green copper pigment and chrysoedla (used in eye shadow) were used on open wounds.

Mesopotamia

Open wounds were washed in milk and water and then dressed with honey or resin; myrrh and frankincense were also used (Forrest 1982). Again, medicine, magic and religion were closely associated.

India

Cauterization
the application of heat sufficient to scar tissue; used to obtain haemostasis

Hindu surgery was already advanced in the first millennium BC, with the famous surgeon Sasruta about 600 BC describing rhinoplasty and the **cauterization** of wounds. The plastic surgical technique described for rhinoplasty was needed because cutting off the nose was a frequent punishment.

Greece

The emphasis for the Greek management of wounds was on hygiene and the use of bland substances. Homer's *Iliad* refers to the Greek army suffering high mortality rates from war injuries.

Influential Individuals

Hippocrates (460–379 BC)

Suppuration
formation of discharge or pus

Hippocrates wrote widely during his lifetime, greatly advancing medicine by describing many diseases. He advocated early haemostasis and the treatment of contused wounds with salves; the purpose of this was to encourage **suppuration**, to debride devitalized tissue and to reduce inflammation (Forrest 1982). Nature, in Hippocrates' opinion, would heal wounds.

Celsus

Nearer to the time of Christ (25 BC–AD 37), Celsus wrote eight books on medicine and surgery. In *De Medicina* Celsus, for the first time, clearly described the four cardinal signs of infection, though these were not specifically describing wounds: '*Nota vera inflammationis sunt quattuor; rubor et tumor cum calor et dolor*' — the signs and symptoms of redness, swelling, heat and pain. Celsus also recommended the early closure of fresh wounds and the surgical debridement of contaminated wounds.

Galen

Pus
a protein-rich liquid which consists of exudate, dead macrophages and bacteria

Aseptic technique
a method of carrying out sterile procedures so that there is the minimum risk of introducing infection. Achieved by the sterility of equipment and a non-touch method.

Towards the end of the Roman era, Galen (AD 129–200), the famous Greek physician and anatomist, wrote around 500 works. His descriptions of routine wound management were typical of treatments of that time. Galen is famous for his theory of 'laudable **pus**', '*pus bonum et laudabile*', advocating that should a wound become infected and suppurate this process should be allowed to continue. Galen believed that when infection localized and then discharged itself the wound would go on to heal without problems. During the Middle Ages medical practitioners misinterpreted this message to mean that pus formation was both desirable and necessary for healthy healing. Clean, uninfected wounds were inoculated with a variety of noxious substances in order to stimulate pus formation. These practices continued from the seventh to the fourteenth centuries. It was not until the nineteenth century that Pasteur and Lister managed to persuade their colleagues that mortality rates could be reduced by using antiseptics and **aseptic** principles.

Paracelsus

Born in 1493, Philippus Aureolus Paracelsus (real name Theophrastus von Hohenheim) developed the theory that man had a juice which continually circulated round the body to keep the tissues and organs healthy and in a good state of repair. Paracelsus taught that all medicines, treatments and dressings should aim to maintain these body juices in the optimum condition. To this end he advocated the use of minerals such as salts of mercury and antimony on wounds. Paracelsus met an unseemly death at the age of 48 in a bar-room brawl, a result of the mixed and colourful company which he kept.

Paré

Ambroise Paré (1510–1593) was the founder of military surgery in the sixteenth century. An advocate of the 'laudable pus' theory, his decision to stop using noxious substances to induce infection came about when the boiling oil he was using on the battlefield ran out and he used, as an alternative, egg yolks on the battle wounds of soldiers. Compared with soldiers treated with boiling oil, soldiers treated with egg yolk had a higher survival rate, and Paré changed his philosophy. Subsequently, Paré said 'I dressed his wounds, God healed him', the quote for which he is famous *'Je le pansay, et Dieu le guarit'*.

Lorenz Heister

Although German, Heister (1683–1758) was most influential in France. Heister described wound treatments, especially the bandages and dressings which were used. He carefully catalogued wounds in great detail, describing their size and shape, and the cocktails of dressings which were used.

Sir Charles Bell

The battle of Waterloo (1815) occurred in an era when advances were being made in surgical technique and the development of surgical instruments. On hearing of the devastation at the battle, Bell travelled to Belgium with his assistant, to find 50 000 dead or injured men. Both sides had suffered terrible injuries and Bell operated on these men 'until his clothes were stiff with blood' and his arms so tired they were 'powerless with exertion of using the knife'. Bell and other surgeons corresponded with each other and, through these letters, it is possible to gain some understanding of the standard of surgery at this time. Surgical **debridement** was a widespread procedure, with devitalized bone and muscle excised. The control of haemorrhage was also undertaken by using ligatures and the range of surgical instruments was quite sophisticated. Many men died of their injuries through sepsis and also tetanus, which would, today, be treatable.

Debridement
the removal of foreign matter or devitalized, injured, infected tissue from a wound until the surrounding healthy tissue is exposed

Louis Pasteur

Pasteur (1822–1895) discovered micro-organisms and bacteria, although initially his interest was not in patients with infection but in the role of bacteria in the fermentation of wines. Pasteur used his knowledge in this field to develop heat sterilization (pasteurization).

Joseph Lister

Joseph Lister (1827–1912) was born to a Quaker family in 1827 and was fortunate to have the high standard of education to which wealthy Quaker families had access. While obtaining a degree in Arts from University College, London, he developed an interest in medicine. His adulthood was hampered by both physical and mental ill-health, and it was not until

1860 that he became a professor of surgery in Glasgow. It was here that Lister worked on aseptic principles, antiseptic treatment of wounds and the use of carbolic spray during surgical procedures. His interest was drawn to the problems related to sepsis and a high mortality rate amongst the patients in the Glasgow hospitals.

Septicaemia
blood poisoning, a systemic disease where pathogenic micro-organisms are present and multiply in the blood. A life-threatening disease

It was Lister who translated Pasteur's work to the field of patient care. Lister used Pasteur's findings to link suppuration of wounds with **septicaemia**, tetanus, gangrene and subsequent death. Although initially Lister used heat sterilization, he soon turned to chemical antiseptics. When Lister discovered how effective carbolic acid was he was able to revolutionize surgical techniques. Infection and mortality rates fell dramatically as Lister used a combination of clean linen, a clean room, the use of carbolic acid spray and hand-washing to reduce infection. Lister was a surgeon in King's College, London, for many years, and for the 2702 patients under his care the post-operative mortality rate was 2%.

Joseph Gamgee

Joseph Gamgee (1828–1886), qualified first as a veterinary surgeon and later studied medicine. He gained experience in the Crimean War and at the Royal Free Hospital in London, going on to work in Birmingham. It was here that Gamgee became interested in wound healing. He wrote of the need for 'utmost gentleness in dealing with wounds and infrequent changes of dressing'. Through working with cotton wool and gauze, he designed an 'absorbent and antiseptic surgical dressing'. This consisted of pads of degreased cotton wool covered in gauze which was bleached to give it absorbency. In these early days this dressing formed a barrier to cross-infection and provided a warm environment at the wound bed. Gamgee also soaked his dressing in phenol and iodine occasionally. Interestingly, gamgee tissue is still available and used today.

The Adoption of Aseptic Techniques

The medical staff of the nineteenth century remained, for many years, unconvinced of the benefits of the principles advocated by Pasteur and Lister. It was only in 1876 that his profession took notice of him when Lister published *On the Antiseptic Principle in the Practice of Surgery*. Gradually his work began to be expanded and developed, with steam sterilization used for surgical instruments and dressings. Theatre and dressing packs became available.

World War I

The introduction of aseptic technique during surgery and the use of operating theatres (as opposed to the kitchen table) brought a more controlled environment to surgery. Scrubbing-up procedures, gloves and sterile dressings were other methods being developed to reduce wound infection.

Tulle gras dressings were developed as a low-adherent dressing. Carbolic acid was found to have too many side-effects so Eusol and Dakin's solution became popular. Eusol (an acronym for Edinburgh University Solution of Lime) contained chlorinated lime and boric acid diluted with water. Dakin's solution contained chlorinated lime, boric acid and sodium carbonate. Infection was a real problem in World War I, with contamination of wounds by earth and dirt being widespread, leading to gas gangrene and many subsequent deaths.

Antibiotics

Alexander Fleming

Through the accidental discovery of penicillin Fleming revolutionized the care of many patients with infections. He found that bactericidal substances were released from *Penicillium* mould. This finding was used in the treatment of humans with infection by Howard Florey and Ernst Chain in 1941.

Leonard Colebrook

At the same time Fleming was working on penicillin, Colebrook was studying the role of haemolytic streptococcus in relation to childbirth and the problems of puerperal sepsis. Colebrook discovered that sulphonamide contained in the dye Prontosil was active against streptococcal infection. Subsequently Colebrook looked at the problem of streptococcal infection in burn patients. Using asepsis and antiseptics, topical penicillin cream and stringent cross-infection measures he much improved the prognosis for burns victims. Due to his political activities the 1952 Fireguard Act was introduced as a way of preventing burns.

The Development of Dressing Materials

The zoologist George Winter (1927–1981) investigated wound healing in cutaneous wounds in the domestic pig. He later became interested in wound dressings and worked on covering wounds in an experimental model (using the pig) and observing healing rates. In his most famous piece of work, Winter observed that wounds covered with an occlusive dressing healed faster than those left to dry out (Winter 1962). It was from this work that the principles of moist wound healing were developed.

Moist Wound Healing

Exudate
wound fluid with a high content of protein and cells that has escaped from blood vessels

Under dry conditions the bed of an open wound rapidly dries out and forms a scab made up of dead and dying cells. New epidermal cells migrate under this scab in the moist environment found under it, so extending the healing phase. In a moist environment **exudate** bathes the wound bed with nutrients, and many modern dressing materials are designed to maintain moisture. In 1985 Turner evaluated the needs of healing wounds and listed the criteria that should be fulfilled by a good wound dressing (Turner 1985):

i)   Maintains high humidity between wound and dressing
ii)   Removes excess exudate and toxic components

iii)   Allows gaseous exchange
iv)   Provides thermal insulation
v)   Impermeable to bacteria
vi)   Free from particles and toxic wound components
vii)   Allows removal without causing trauma during dressing change

This was further expanded in 1990 when Thomas evaluated the functions of a dressing (Thomas 1990b). Dressings should ensure that the wound remains:

i)   Moist with exudate, but not macerated
ii)   Free of clinical infection and excessive slough
iii)   Free of toxic chemicals, particles or fibres released by the dressing
iv)   At the optimal temperature for healing to take place
v)   Undisturbed by frequent or unnecessary dressing changes
vi)   At an optimum pH value

Later, Morison (1992) provided a nursing perspective of criteria for an ideal wound dressing:

i)   Non-adherent
ii)   Impermeable to bacteria
iii)   Capable of maintaining a high humidity at the wound site while removing excess exudate
iv)   Thermally insulating
v)   Non-toxic and non-allergenic
vi)   Comfortable and conformable
vii)   Capable of protecting the wound from further trauma
viii)   Requires infrequent dressing changes
ix)   Cost-effective
x)   Long shelf-life
xi)   Available both in hospital and in the community

The range of modern wound dressings is outlined in Table 3.1, which lists their properties, presentation, dressing change frequency and indications. Examples of many of these dressings in use are shown in Figures 3.1 to 3.7.

Management of Sutured Wounds

The vast majority of sutured wounds heal without complication. Dressings applied in theatre need not be changed or disturbed unless there is a good reason for doing so. Dressings should be changed and the incision site observed if:

i)   the dressings become stained by discharge
ii)   the clinical signs of infection are present, i.e. pain, inflammation, redness, impaired movement
iii)   the patient shows general signs of infection

Table 3.1 *The range of modern wound dressings*

Dressing	Properties	Availability	Dressing change frequency	Indications
Semipermeable film e.g. Opsite, Tegaderm	Self-adhesive films, see-through for easy observation of the wound Conformable and resistant to shear and tear Vapour permeable	Sheets ranging from 5 cm × 5 cm to very large drapes for theatre use	Designed to stay in place for several days Should be changed when leakage is imminent, or has occurred	Superficial and epithelializing wounds: minor burns, skin graft donor sites, grades I and II pressure sores Postoperative dressing for sutured wounds IV line sites
Low-adherent e.g. Melolin, Telfa, N-A Dressing, Tegapore	Some absorbency and low adherence to wound bed Textile dressings allow wound exudate to pass through dressing	Sheets of various sizes from 5 cm × 5 cm	When saturated or for wound observation	Wounds producing little exudate or as a primary contact material with additional padding
Multilayer e.g. Spirosorb, Spiroflex	Absorbent and self-adherent Conformable	Sheets	When saturated, leaking or for wound observation	Low to moderately exuding wounds of all types
Medicated low-adherent dressings e.g. Inadine, Iodoflex, Actisorb Plus	Low-adherent dressings which deliver antiseptics, so used as bactericidal dressings	Sheets	When saturated, leaking or when active agent absorbed (could be daily)	Wound beds with superficial wound infection, especially *Pseudomonas* (iodine) and broad-spectrum (Actisorb Plus)
Alginates (pure calcium or calcium and sodium) e.g. Sorbsan, Tegagel	Absorbent; when absorbing exudate forms a hydrophilic gel Haemostatic (Kaltostat)	Flat sheets of various sizes Rope packing Also with films and extra padding	When saturated Often can stay in place for several days	Exuding wounds of many aetiologies, especially heavily exuding wounds Packing useful for irregular-shaped cavities and those with undermining and sinuses
Foams e.g. Allevyn, Allevyn CWD, Cavicare, Lyofoam, Lyofoam E	Absorbent Some brands more absorbent than others Some sheets self-adherent	Flat sheet, cavity dressing	When saturated Can stay in place for several days	Exuding wounds of all aetiologies Cavicare cannot be used in sinuses or wounds that undermine the skin edges
Hydrocolloids e.g. Comfeel, Granuflex, Tegasorb	Absorbent, forms a soft gel Sheets are self-adherent Occlusive or semi-occlusive	Flat sheets, powders, paste, gel	When saturated, as indicated by imminent leakage or leakage Designed to stay intact for 4–5 days	Exuding wounds, especially chronic Can facilitate autolysis of devitalized tissue from the wound bed
Hydrogels e.g. Intrasite, Granugel	Maintains a very moist environment Often used in conjunction with a semipermeable film	Single use applications	To facilitate wound debridement daily To maintain moisture on slightly exuding wounds, can be left for 2–3 days	Most efficient at achieving wound debridement Moist environment facilitates autolysis of devitalized tissue from the wound bed Can also be used as a cavity filler
Pads and absorbent cottons e.g. AD pads, gamgee roll	Absorbent	A variety of sizes	When saturated	As secondary dressing to provide extra absorbency or additional padding to protect the wounded area

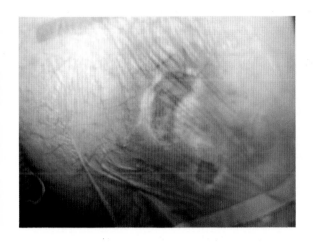

Figure 3.1 *A semipermeable film dressing being used to treat a stage II pressure sore.*

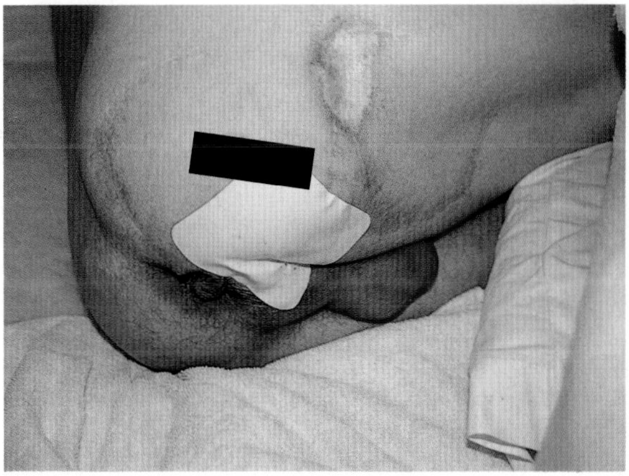

Figure 3.2 *An adhesive foam dressing being used in the anal area to prevent wound contamination.*

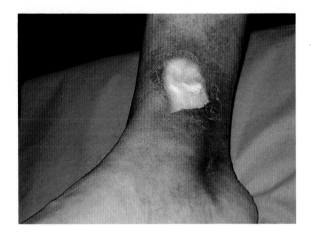

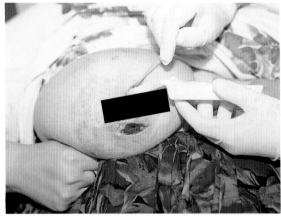

Figure 3.3 *An alginate dressing used as a primary wound contact on a venous leg ulcer prior to compression therapy.*

Figure 3.4 *An alginate rope being packed into a cavity wound.*

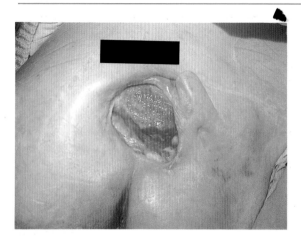
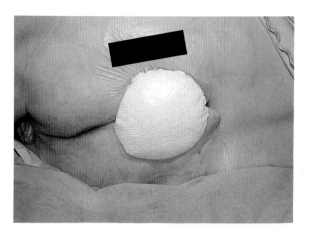

Figure 3.5   *Hydrocellular foam dressing used on a heavily exuding sacral pressure sore (left). The dressing is held in place with a semipermeable film (right).*

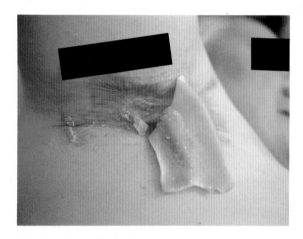
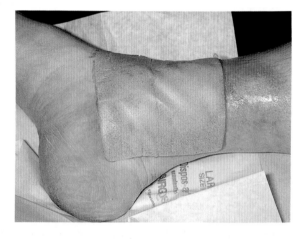

Figure 3.6   *A hydrocolloid dressing following four days treatment on an axillary wound.*

Figure 3.7   *A hydrocolloid dressing used as a primary wound contact for a venous leg ulcer.*

Management of Open or Granulating Wounds

Debridement of Devitalized Tissue

The presence of sloughy, necrotic, devitalized tissue on the wound bed can delay healing and also increases the risk of wound infection (Figure 3.8). It is important to remove devitalized tissue as quickly and efficiently as possible. This can be difficult to achieve, however, as both slough and necrotic tissue

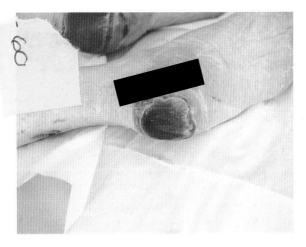

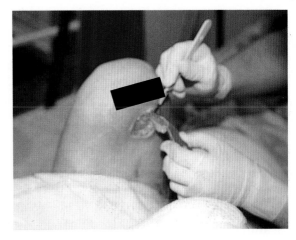

Figure 3.8 *Necrotic tissue on the bed of a pressure sore. It may have deep tissue damage underneath.*

Figure 3.9 *Surgical debridement of necrotic tissue.*

are firmly stuck to the wound bed and cannot simply be wiped away. There are several ways of achieving wound debridement.

Surgical debridement

Surgical debridement is by far the quickest and most effective method as debridement is immediate and a healthy wound bed can result (Figure 3.9). However, thorough and effective surgical debridement down to healthy, viable tissue is best undertaken by a doctor with surgical skills, as some bleeding usually results. For some patients access to a surgeon is not possible, especially when patients are being cared for in the community.

The use of modern dressing materials

Hydrogels and **hydrocolloids** effectively rehydrate devitalized tissue. In the presence of sufficient moisture, **autolysis** of devitalized tissue takes place. With prolonged use of moist dressings the autolytic processes will facilitate separation of viable from non-viable tissue. Eventually the sloughy or necrotic tissue becomes soft and can be gently cut off the wound bed.

Chemical debridement

Chemicals such as hypochlorites have, in the past, been recommended to effect debridement. Experimental trials conducted by Thomas (1990a), however, found hypochlorites to be ineffective for this purpose. Thomas found that about 100 ml of 0.25% chlorine solution is needed to solubilize only 1 g of sloughy tissue. Thomas also immersed necrotic tissue in Eusol and showed that after 24 hours this tissue remained unchanged.

Hydrogel
a dressing material which consists of a water-containing gel

Hydrocolloid
a dressing material made up of a colloid in which water is the dispersion medium

Autolysis
the breakdown of devitalized tissues. The disintegration of cells or tissues by endogenous enzymes

Enzymatic agents

Globally, several enzymatic agents are available as debriding agents. In the UK a preparation containing a mixture of streptokinase and streptodornase (Varidase) is available. Some caution should be exercised, however, when using this product. When the wound bed consists of a thick, dry **eschar**, enzymatic agents have been found to be ineffective (Hellgren 1983). Some practitioners have recommended that, in this situation, Varidase may be injected under the eschar (Morison 1992), although this procedure should be carried out only by experienced practitioners (Thomas 1990a).

Eschar
dead, devitalized tissue

Healthy Granulating and Epithelializing Wounds

The aim of intervention for wounds that are in the proliferative phase of healing and producing granulation tissue is to maintain an environment for healing. Following assessment of the patient, the wound characteristics and the social environment of the patient, a nursing model can be selected and a wound care plan formulated.

Excessive Exudate Production

Although exudate is produced by all healthy open wounds, excessive exudate may be produced by particularly large wounds or deep cavities. If exudate is not controlled, leakage may occur which soils and stains clothes and bed-clothes, so causing discomfort and embarrassment. Excessive exudate can also cause maceration to the skin surrounding the wound. Exudate can be controlled by using absorbent dressing materials (e.g. **alginates** and hydrophilic foams) and by frequent dressing changes.

Alginates
a group of wound dressings derived from seaweed

Excessive Granulation Tissue (Proud Flesh)

Granulation tissue can be produced in excessive amounts and rise above the level of the skin. Epithelium will not cover this tissue and intervention is required to flatten the wound surface and so facilitate re-epithelialization. Several treatments are available including the application of silver nitrate sticks (75%) and corticosteroid cream. A small study using a flat foam dressing (Harris and Rolstad 1993) found this an effective method of controlling excessive granulation tissue.

Managing Wound Infection

Management of wound infection presents nurses with difficult challenges. Prevention of wound infection related to the physical hospital environment may be achieved by:

i)   Ensuring that adequate space is maintained between the beds of patients. Where insufficient space is available, particularly in an open ward, the wound infection rate increases. Bibby *et al.* (1986) found an increased wound infection rate where open wards accommodated more than 25 patients.

ii)   Reducing the time between admission and operation to a minimum. Using preadmission clinics and day surgery units is one way of achieving this. The longer the patient is in hospital, the greater the chance of colonization by the pathogenic bacteria found in hospital.

iii) Only prepare patient's skin in theatre, or stop shaving skin altogether. The lowest clean wound infection rate is 0.9% where patients are not shaved pre-operatively, compared with 2.5% when patients are shaved (Spencer and Bale 1990).

iv) Reduce time spent operating as much as possible. The prolonging of time spent operating increases the risk of infection in clean wounds (Cruse and Foord 1973).

v) Avoid contamination at the time of operation. An infection rate of 1–2% is expected in clean, elective operations, compared with 40% in emergency, contaminated surgery (Westaby and White 1985).

vi) Avoid the use of drains as this increases the risk of wound infection. Where drains cannot be avoided a closed drainage system results in less wound infection than an open drainage system (Cruse and Foord 1973).

vii) Using good hand-washing techniques.

Where wound infection has developed the management of the individual will depend on a number of factors.

Management of Patients with MRSA-positive Wound Swabs

i) Screen patients fully (i.e. swab axillae, nose, throat and perineum) and treat with mupirocin ointment 2% topically for 10 days only.

ii) Apply mupirocin daily to the wound bed

iii) Swab at weekly intervals following treatment. The patient is considered clear when three consecutive negative swabs have been obtained.

iv) Where topical mupirocin is not effective, consider using a short course of rifampicin systemically together with another antibiotic to which the strain is sensitive (Duckworth 1993).

v) Where patients have a serious infection vancomycin can be administered intravenously.

Localized Wound Infection

Sutured wounds which develop a localized infection often discharge spontaneously, so draining the infection. It may be necessary to remove one or two sutures to facilitate complete drainage (Figures 3.10 to 3.12). A specimen of pus can be sent for culture and sensitivity if antibiotic therapy is being considered. Once the pus has been drained a packing material such as an alginate rope can be inserted into the wound to maintain drainage and allow the wound to heal from its depths.

When drainage of the abscess is not complete, surgical incision may be required, especially if the abscess is deep-seated; again, a dressing is used to ensure sound healing from the base of the wound (Figures 3.13 and 3.14).

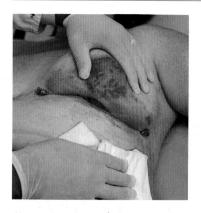

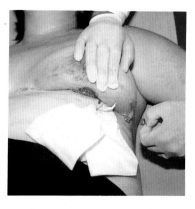

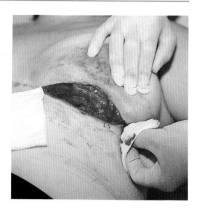

Figure 3.10   *A patient 10 days following reduction mammoplasty showing signs of gross wound infection.*

Figure 3.11   *Removing the suture to release pus and infected fluid.*

Figure 3.12   *The resultant cavity wound.*

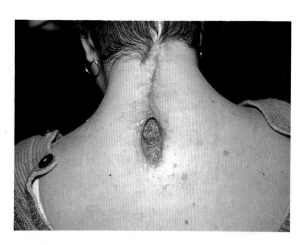

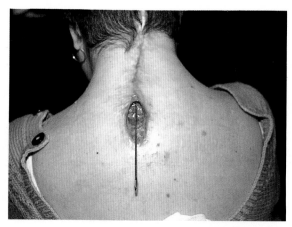

Figure 3.13   *Wound prior to assessment.*

Figure 3.14   *Following probing, a large cavity is detected under the suture line.*

Infection in Open Granulating Wounds

Following assessment and the results of bacteriological culture and sensitivity, it may be appropriate either to treat the patient with systemic antibiotics or to apply local antiseptics to the wound bed to eradicate the pathogen causing the wound infection.

While a wound infection persists it may be wise to perform more frequent wound cleansing, in an attempt to reduce the bacterial count at the wound bed.

Aseptic Techniques

Employing aseptic technique to prevent wound infection

Use of an aseptic technique is aimed at preventing micro-organisms coming into contact with a wound from the nurse, the environment or the patient.

Although the principles of asepsis and cross-contamination are clear, traditionally the technique was taught as a rigid procedure with little room for nurses to adapt it to individual situations. Lack of knowledge of the underlying principles often resulted in nurses using the technique unnecessarily in certain circumstances, or cutting the wrong corners when time or resources were scarce. As little research has been carried out in this area, nurses have little supporting evidence on which to make decisions about when to employ a strict aseptic technique or a socially clean procedure.

The indications for the type of procedure to use can be rationalized by considering the mode of bacterial spread and the type of wound being dealt with.

Reducing the spread of bacteria by the non-touch technique

Aseptic technique has been synonymous with use of forceps, cotton wool and the 'clean' and 'dirty' hand method (Kelso 1989). Forceps can cause harm to delicate healing tissue, and Thomlinson (1987) demonstrated that a non-touch technique was adequately achieved with gloved hands or hands washed in chlorhexidine (Hibisol).

Swabbing the wound with cotton wool or even gauze can provide a direct route for bacterial growth by shedding fibres into granulating tissue (Wood 1976, Archer 1990). Cleaning, if required at all, is best carried out by irrigation (see below), as swabbing the wound only results in organisms being redistributed around the wound.

The clean and dirty hand method has also little to support its continued practice. Again, it undermines the underlying principles of asepsis, as hand-washing and the use of gloves are sufficient precautions to avoid contamination of the wound.

The nurse should be aware of what constitutes 'clean' and 'dirty'. Having removed a dirty dressing with a gloved hand or a disposable bag, both should be disposed of before commencing the now clean procedure. Between the 'clean' and 'dirty' procedures, rinsing hands with alcoholic disinfectant should be sufficient (Gould 1987).

Application of basic principles such as use of gloves, hand-washing, wound irrigation and sterile dressings can be adapted both to the hospital patient in a surgical ward with an acute wound and to the patient nursed at home with chronic leg ulcers.

Wearing gloves should never replace scrupulous hand-washing, but is an essential precaution when the skin is broken, as transmission of blood-borne viruses such as human immunodeficiency virus (HIV) is possible through damaged skin (Gurevich 1989).

Hand-washing

The most effective method of preventing cross-infection is to use a good hand-washing technique. As with the rest of the skin, hands carry bacteria which are permanently resident and which can only be eradicated for a few hours. However, the skin can also be contaminated with transient pathogenic organisms which are picked up and then shed. It is possible to remove these pathogenic organisms by adequate hand-washing (Gould 1987). Although many healthcare professionals, nurses included, profess to be knowledgeable about the importance of good hand-washing, few practise the technique (McFarlene 1992). The thoroughness of the hand-washing depends on the task to be done:

- Social hand-washing is undertaken when starting work, finishing work, before meal breaks, after using the lavatory, and when visiting other wards and departments. Soap and water is adequate for this purpose.
- Hygienic hand-washing is undertaken before invasive procedures, after contact with infected patients, after procedures involving high-risk patients and after handling contaminated equipment. An antiseptic hand-washing agent is used.
- Surgical hand-washing is undertaken in preparation for surgical procedures. A 3-minute hand-washing procedure using an antiseptic agent is required.

Basic hand-washing technique
Using running water and either soap or antiseptic wash, five strokes forward and five strokes backwards are used for each of the following steps (Ayliffe *et al.* 1978):

(a)   Palm to palm
(b)   Right palm over left dorsum and left palm over right dorsum
(c)   Palm to palm with fingers interlaced
(d)   Backs of fingers to opposing palms with fingers interlaced
(e)   Rotational rubbing of right thumb clasped over left palm and left thumb over right palm
(f)   Rotational rubbing backwards and forwards with clasped fingers of right hand in palm of left hand and vice versa
(g)   Hands and wrists rubbed for 30 seconds

Thorough drying of hands should follow (McFarlene 1992).

These steps may be difficult to follow. The makers of antiseptic agents

Figure 3.15
*Handwashing technique –
see text for more details.
(From Ayliffe et al. 1978;
Lawrence 1985.)*

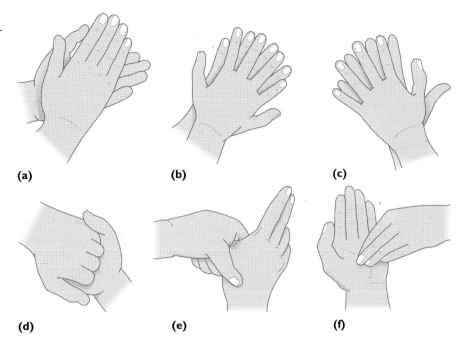

(a)   (b)   (c)

(d)   (e)   (f)

have produced pictures of these steps which can be pinned over sinks to assist in hand-washing (Figure 3.15).

Wound Cleansing

Colonization
the presence of commensal
or pathogenic organisms
which multiply on the
wound but do not cause
infection

Routine cleansing of wounds is still practised in many areas of wound care (Roe *et al.* 1994, Jones *et al.* 1995). Nurses still do not question exactly what they are trying to achieve by cleansing a wound every time they change a dressing. Indications for cleansing are clear if the underlying principles of wound healing and bacterial **colonization** are understood. The following points should be borne in mind before cleansing procedures are undertaken.

Removal of wound exudate

Normal wound repair requires the bactericidal activity and growth factors present in the inflammatory exudate (Hohn *et al.* 1977; Chen *et al.* 1992). Removal of wound fluid through cleansing and then drying of the wound may only deplete the healing tissue of these vital components and contradicts the principles of moist wound healing.

Elimination of bacteria on the wound surface

It is often believed that cleansing will eliminate harmful bacteria from the wound (Thomlinson 1987). It is not possible or even advisable (Johnson 1988) to remove all bacteria from the wound surface. Furthermore, as

Thomlinson's study demonstrated, attempts to cleanse surgical wounds only succeed in distributing pathogenic organisms along the suture line.

Indications for cleansing

Wounds should only be cleansed to remove excess exudate, slough or necrotic tissue and remnants of old dressing material, all of which can become a focus for infection. However, wounds caused by accidental trauma often contain large amounts of debris and are grossly contaminated, and these require thorough cleansing (Dire *et al.* 1990). Patients with thermal injuries also require wound cleansing because the wound is at greater risk of infection, being no longer colonized with normal flora (Lawrence 1991).

Types of cleansing fluid

Although antiseptic solutions were widely used in the past, their usage is mainly limited to accident and emergency departments (Jones *et al.* 1995), where it is hoped that these solutions will have an antibacterial effect on grossly contaminated wounds. However, most antiseptics are rapidly inactivated by body fluids and therefore not in contact long enough to succeed in killing bacteria (Ferguson 1988). Studies have shown that antiseptics can be harmful to healing tissue (Deas *et al.* 1986; Leaper 1988), but it must be remembered that these laboratory studies were performed on animals and have yet to be replicated on human wounds.

Cleansing can be adequately achieved, even in traumatic wounds, with the use of normal saline. Studies have also demonstrated that there is no increased risk of infection when sutured wounds are washed with soap and water (Noe and Keller 1988) or when the patient showers (Chrintz *et al.* 1989). Chronic wounds such as leg ulcers can equally well be cleansed with ordinary tap-water (Lawrence 1991).

Method of cleansing

As already described, swabbing a wound with cotton wool or gauze swabs is inadvisable and probably ineffective. Where large amounts of fluid are required to remove debris this is best achieved by irrigation. It can be difficult to judge the amount of pressure to use without damaging underlying tissue. Gentle irrigation for normal cleansing can be achieved with use of a syringe or quill, or a jug of warmed saline. When water is used, immersing the wound area in a bowl or bath may be an easy way to remove debris or exudate and less painful to the patient (Figures 3.16 and 3.17).

Care must be taken, especially in the hospital environment, that baths, bowls or lifting equipment are cleansed properly between patient use (Ayliffe 1988).

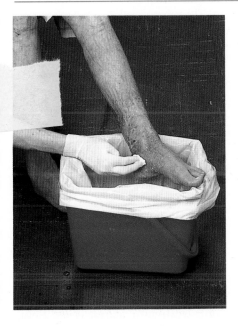

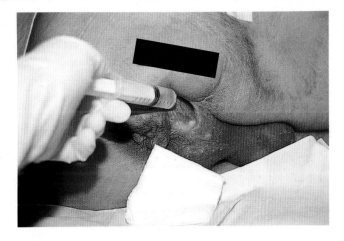

Figure 3.17 *Wound irrigation in a difficult area to treat. This pressure sore was irrigated with normal saline using a syringe.*

Figure 3.16 *Wound cleansing for a patient with leg ulceration. A bin liner has been used to prevent contamination of the bucket.*

Conclusion

Cleansing of a wound should only be performed when clearly indicated, and irrigation with saline or water should in most cases be sufficient. Wounds that are clean, with healthy tissue, do not require cleansing and should be left undisturbed to maintain an optimum environment for healing.

Summary

Although wound interventions are becoming more and more sophisticated, the basis of managing any wound successfully has been outlined in this chapter.

Before moving on to the case studies section ensure that you have understood the following basic principles:

- The development of dressing materials:
    moist wound healing
    range of modern dressings
- Management of sutured and granulating wounds:
    signs of infection
    debridement of devitalized tissue
    exudate production
- Prevention of infection:
    aseptic technique
    hand-washing

- Wound cleansing
  indications for cleansing
  methods of cleansing

Further Reading

Cockbill SME (1992) Wound care problems in the community. In: *Proceedings of the First European Conference on Advances in Wound Management.* London: Macmillan.

Freshwater D (1992) Pre-operative preparation of the skin — a review of the literature. *Surgical Nurse* 5(5): 6–10.

Leaper DJ & Lucarotti ME (1992) Sutures and staples. *Journal of Wound Care* 1(4): 27–30.

David JA (1986) *Wound Management: A Comprehensive Guide to Dressing and Healing.* London: Martin Dunitz.

Turner TD & Stevens P (1982) Which dressing and why? *Nursing Times Wound Care* 11 (July): 41–44.

Forrest RD (1982) Early history of wound treatment. *Journal of the Royal Society of Medicine* 75: 198–205.

Thomas S (1992) *Wound Management and Dressing.* London: Pharmaceutical Press.

Moore D (1992) Hypochlorites: a review of the evidence. *Journal of Wound Care* 1(4): 44–49.

Ayliffe, GAS, Lowbury EJL, Geddes AM & Williams JD (eds) (1992) Control of Hospital Infection, 3rd edn. London: Chapman & Hall.

Morison M (1991) A Colour Guide to the Nursing Management of Wounds. London: Wolfe.

References

Archer HA (1990) A controlled model of moist wound healing. *Journal of Experimental Pathology* 71: 155–170.

Ayliffe GAJ (1988) Equipment-related infection risks. *Journal of Hospital Infection* (supplement A) 11: 279–284.

Ayliffe GAJ, Babb JR & Cenoraishi AH (1978) A test for hygienic hand disinfection.

Bergmark M (1967) *Vallort och Vitlok: om Folkmedicinens Lakeorter Natur od Kultur.* Stockholm.

Bibby BA, Colling GS & Ayliffe G (1986) A mathematical model for assessing the risk of post-operative wound infection. *Journal of Hospital Infection* 8: 31–38.

Chen WY, Rogers AA & Lydon MJ (1992) Characterization of biologic properties of wound fluid collected during early stages of wound healing. *Journal of Investigative Dermatology,* 99(5): 559–564.

Chrintz H, Vibits H, Cordtz TO *et al.* (1989) Need for surgical wound dressing. *British Journal of Surgery* 76: 204–205.

Cruse PJE & Foord R (1973) A five year prospective study of 23 649 surgical wounds. *Archives of Surgery* 107: 206–271.

Deas J, Billings P, Brennan SS, Silver I & Leaper DJ (1986) The toxicity of commonly used antiseptics on fibroblasts in tissue culture. *Phlebology* 1: 205–209.

Dire D, Hood F & Welsh A (1990) A comparison of wound irrigation solutions used in the emergency department. *Annals of Emergency Medicine* 19: 143–147.

Duckworth G (1993) Diagnosis and management of methicillin-resistant *Staphylococcus aureus* infection. *British Medical Journal* 307: 1049–1052.

Ferguson A (1988) Best performer. *Nursing Times* 84(14): 52–55.

Forrest RD (1982) Early history of wound treatment. *Journal of Royal Society of Medicine* 75: 198–205.

Gould D (1987) *Infection and Patient Care*. London: Heinemann.

Gurevich I (1989) Aids in critical care: realistic concerns and appropriate precautions. *Heart and Lung* 18(2): 107–112.

Harris A & Rolstad BS (1993) Hypergranulation tissue a non-traumatic method of management. In: Harding KG, Cherry G & Turner TD (eds) *Proceedings of the Second European Conference on Advances in Wound Management*. London: Macmillan.

Hellgren L (1983) Cleansing properties of stabilised trypsin and streptokinase-streptodornase in necrotic leg ulcers. *European Journal of Clinical Pharmacology* 24: 623–628.

Hohn DC, Ponce B, Burton RW & Hunt TK (1977) Antimicrobial systems of the surgical wound. *American Journal of Surgery* 113: 597–600.

Johnson A (1988) The cleansing ethic. *Community Outlook* Feb, 8–10.

Jones V, Bale, S & Harding KG (1995) Assessment of Wound Cleansing. *Proceedings of the Fourth European Conference on Advances in Wound Management*, London: Macmillan.

Kelso H (1989) Alternative technique. The Journal of Infection Control Nursing Supplement. *Nursing Times* 85(23): 70–72.

Knight B (1985) The history of wound treatment in wound care. In: Westaby S (ed.) *Wound Care*. London: Heinemann.

Lawrence C (1991) Bacterial infection of wounds. *Wound Management* 1: 13–15.

Leaper DJ (1986) The wound healing process. In: Turner TD, Schmidt RS & Harding KG (eds) *Advances in Wound Management*. Chichester: John Wiley.

Leaper D & Camerson S (1988) Antiseptic toxicity in open wounds. *Nursing Times* 84(25): 77–79.

McFarlene A (1992) Why do we forget to remember hand washing. In: Harne EM & Cowan T (eds) *Staff Nurses' Survival Guide*. London: Wolfe.

Morison M (1992) Priorities in wound management: which dressing? In: *A Colour Guide to the Nursing Management of Wounds*, pp. 33–47. London: Wolfe.

Noe JM & Keller M (1988) Can stitches get wet? *Plasic and Reconstructive Surgery* 82: 205.

Roe BH, Griffiths JM, Kenrick M *et al.* (1994) Nursing treatment of patients with chronic leg ulcers in the community. *Journal of Clinical Nursing* 3: 159–168.

Spencer K & Bale S (1990) A logical approach: management of surgical wounds. *Professional Nurse* 5(6): 303–306.

Thomas S (1990a) Eusol revisited. *Dressing Times* 3: 1.

Thomas S (1990b) Functions of a wound dressing. In: *Wound Management and Dressings*. London: Pharmaceutical Press.

Thomlinson D (1987) To clean or not to clean. *Nursing Times* 83: 71–75.

Turner TD (1985) Semiocclusive and occlusive dressings. In: Ryan TJ (ed.) *An Environment for Healing: the Role of Occlusion*, pp. 6–14. Royal Society of Medicine Congress and Symposium Series 8, London: RSM.

Westaby S & White S (1985) Wound infection. In: Westaby S (ed.) *Wound Care*. London: Heinemann.

Winter GD (1962) Formation of the scab and rate of epithelialisation of superficial wounds in the skin of the young domestic pig. *Nature* 193: 293–294.

Wood RA (1976) Disintegration of cellulose dressings in open granulating wounds. *British Medical Journal* 1: 1444–1445.

4

Wound Care in the Baby and Young Child

Key issues

This is the first of the life-cycle chapters and deals with the neonate, baby and young child.

Clinical Case Studies

Illustrate the aetiology and management of:

- Extravasation injury
- The rare genetic disorder of histiocytosis X
- Purpuric rash of meningococcal meningitis
- Thermal injury caused by a scald
- Traumatic injury caused by a dog-bite

Nursing Models

Examples of their application to practice are taken from:

- Riehl's interaction model
- Roy's adaptation model
- Peplau's model

Practice points

As you read through this chapter concentrate on the following:

- the choice of dressings that will alleviate pain, minimize trauma and scarring
- the size and type of dressing suitable for babies and small children
- the ways in which nurses can interact with parents and children to decrease emotional trauma
- the importance of documentation of the wound, however small

Introduction

In infants the neonatal period covers the first 4 weeks of life. When considering the whole life-cycle the neonatal period is the most hazardous, with mortality being high. The neonatal mortality rate is defined as the number of liveborn infants who die before the age of 28 days per 1000 births in the same year. Although infant mortality in the UK has fallen from 117.1 in 1910 to 10.8 in 1982, the fall in neonatal mortality has been less dramatic, falling from 40.2 in 1910 to 6.2 in 1982. For neonates the first day of life is vital — more neonates die on their first day than during the life-cycle period from 12 months to 25 years. It follows that caring for neonates and infants with wounds presents nurses with many difficult problems. The most obvious is the smallness and the vulnerability of the neonate. In babies born prematurely this is even more pronounced.

The young child with a wound and wound problems also has special requirements. This is a challenging area of nursing and one in which the creativity and skills of the nurse can be decisive in producing the best possible outcome for the child. The principles of caring for sick children must be considered in conjunction with all the principles of managing patients with wounds as previously discussed.

The principles of managing sick children are dealt with only in relation to issues specific to wound management. Further reading on the management of sick children can be found in paediatric nursing textbooks (see Further Reading).

Nursing Infants

Where serious illness of an infant occurs the family is often thrown into physical and emotional crisis. With support many stable families are able to cope, though less stable ones may experience great difficulties. The paediatric ward staff are highly trained in understanding the needs of, and in caring for, the whole family when an infant is admitted to hospital. On admission the immediate goals of the staff include:

i)   Gaining the parents' cooperation and trust
ii) Alleviating anxiety or restoring it to an acceptable level
iii) Preserving the relationships between the parent and infant (Mead 1991)

 Nurses achieve these goals by:

i)   Explaining all the medical and nursing procedures and by enlisting the help and support of parents to promote a feeling of partnership between staff and parents
ii) Encouraging parents to stay with their baby for as long as possible, or to visit at any time of the day or night (it is usual for beds or chairs to be provided for parents at the infant's bedside, so that they need not be separated)
iii) Helping the parents to understand that regression often occurs. Boredom can also be a problem for infants. This can be helped by placing interesting toys near the child, by talking and interacting with the child whenever they are close, and by allowing siblings and other older children to play with or around the child.

One of the main principles of nursing sick children is to meet he needs of the child as an individual. This involves:

- Recognizing each child as a unique, developing individual whose best interests must be paramount
- Listening to children, attempting to understand their perspectives, opinions and feelings and acknowledging their right to privacy
- Considering the physical, psychological, social, cultural and spiritual needs of the children and their families
- Respecting the right of children, according to their age and understanding, to appropriate information and informed participation in decisions about their care (RCN 1992)

A child may have a wound for a variety of reasons and can easily misunderstand the nature of the wound, why it is there and how it will heal. The role of the child's family is an important factor in planning the wound care of an individual child. As healthcare is shared with the family, the parents especially become actively involved in delivering wound care to their child. Although it is important to recognize that not all parents will want to become actively involved, the majority can feel happy and comfortable about delivering basic wound care to their child. The nurse in this situation provides the education and support which enables parents to learn the necessary skills.

Children feel more confident when it is their parents who provide as much of their wound care as possible. Children also need little encouragement in taking part, often in removing surgical tape and dressings and in cleansing their own wounds. The physical surroundings in hospital make a huge difference to the attitude of the child. Children's wards, accident and emergency departments and haematology units, for example, usually provide facilities separate from those of adults which are appropriate to the needs of children.

Pain

Assessment of a child's pain and the subsequent effective management of that pain can be extremely difficult. Pain has been defined in numerous and complex ways but at the end of the day pain is 'whatever the patient says it is, and exists whenever he says it does' (McCaffery and Beebe 1989).

Historically, the attitudes to children's experiences of pain are interesting. Although much research had been undertaken on pain in the adult, it was not until the 1970s that pain was considered to be an important issue in paediatrics (Melforth 1995).

Children may have difficulties in expressing and communicating to others that they are experiencing pain and also in describing what sort of pain they have (Llewellyn 1994). With careful observation nurses and parents can help assess a child's pain in three ways:

i)   By listening carefully to the child; young children may use a variety of different phrases to express that they are in pain, whereas older children can be quite specific

ii) By observing changes in the child's behaviour (the parent may report such changes)

iii) The child may show physiological signs of pain such as increased pulse rate, blood pressure and respiratory rate

Wound management, including dressing changes, need not be associated with pain or discomfort. The nurses' skill in assessing the child with a wound should ensure that the most appropriate wound treatment and dressing is chosen to minimize trauma at dressing changes.

Dressings Suitable for Children

In hospital the ward nurse can support and encourage the parents to learn to care for the child's wound. Once the child is home the community nurse is able to continue this support. The child may wish to return to school, nursery or more normal activity before the wound is completely healed. A range of dressing materials are available to meet the needs of children with different wound types and problems. The choice of dressing and wound care needs to be a joint decision between the child, parents and nurse. Certain dressing materials are particularly suitable for children, especially those which provide an occlusive or semiocclusive environment. As discussed in Chapter 3, these materials include semipermeable films and hydrocolloids which are self-adherent and isolate the wound from the outside environment. The child is thus able to play and bathe without the parents having to worry about the wound getting dirty or wet. For deeper, cavity wounds semi-permeable films can be used to hold other dressing materials in place, for example alginates, gels and foams.

Caution is needed when applying topical agents to large areas in the neonate, as absorption (for example of calcium from alginates) may interfere with their delicate electrolyte balance. The majority of modern dressing materials are soft, conformable and comfortable, and come in a wide range of sizes so that small children are well catered for.

Wound cleansing and dressing application

It can be extremely difficult to perform a strict aseptic technique on a baby or small child. Small children are easily distracted and get bored, and also may be frightened by a dressing pack and equipment. Even using gloves can cause some children great distress. Hands cleansed with chlorhexidine can be used for wound dressing and dressing changes either by a parent or the nurse (Tomlinson 1987). As an alternative, the use of a shower head or bowl of water may provide a less frightening alternative to wound irrigation with a syringe and quill. As with adults, wound cleansing and dressing changes should only be carried out when indicated. Such indications include the presence of devitalized tissue, infection or excess exudate production. Unnecessary, repeated wound cleansing and dressing changes will only traumatize newly forming tissue.

Returning to normal activity

Wound therapies and dressing should permit the child to have as near normal day-to-day activities as possible. To facilitate this the nurse may choose dressing materials that are not bulky, or use items of clothing to hold dressings in place. In small babies, napkins can be used to hold dressings in the perineal area in place. Children may also pull or fiddle with their dressings, and it may be necessary to apply a pad and bandage over the top of this.

Extravasation Injury

Extravasation injuries may occur as a consequence of the difficulty of giving intravenous fluids to small children. Case Study 4.1 describes a typical problem.

Case Study 4.1
Extravasation injury

Ten-day-old Samantha Marks was born at 40 weeks' gestation and is a well-developed full term neonate. Following a normal delivery, Samantha was progressing well until 5 days after delivery she became restless and irritable, refusing to feed, and was found to be pyrexic (38 °C). Microbiological examination revealed that she had a gram-negative septicaemia which was immediately treated with a course of intravenous antibiotics, via an infusion which was sited in her left foot.

During infusion the cannula became dislodged and a large amount of antibiotic solution invaded the subcutaneous tissue of her foot. The infusion was resited in the right foot, but the damage to the left foot resulted in an area of inflamed tissue which extended over the whole of the dorsal area.

Initially treated with dry dressing by the paediatric nurses, within 3 days the inflamed area became necrotic and sloughy, exuding large amounts of exudate, and inflammation began to spread up Samantha's leg. The area was obviously very painful when touched and, although her general condition was now improving, the wound was causing Samantha and her parents great distress (Figure 4.1).

Aetiology

In neonates an infusion may be sited in the scalp and foot as cannulation in the cubital fossae or hands is technically difficult. During illness some infants will require fluids to be given intravenously. Infants have a higher fluid requirement in proportion to their surface area than adults, and during illness the basal metabolic rate can significantly increase. In infants the

Figure 4.1
Extravasation injury.

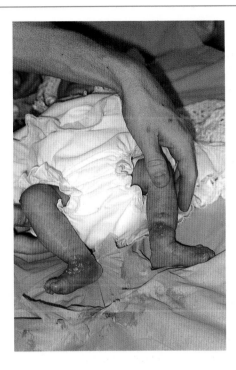

kidneys are immature and so fluid intake must be closely monitored. Intravenous infusions are often given into scalp and foot veins in very small infants. Extravasation injuries are often the result of intravenous solutions leaking into the surrounding tissue. Infiltration of fluid may result in scarring or amputation with fatal consequences (Young 1995). A higher percentage of injuries occur when sited in lower limbs and, in some situations, damage occurs to the nerves and tendons, with ensuing tissue death and necrosis.

Management

Should extravasation occur, the infusion must be stopped immediately, the cannula removed, the doctor advised, and the pharmacist contacted to advise on the potential toxicity of the infused substance. Prevention of this type of tissue injury can be best achieved by frequent observation of the infusion site. It is therefore advisable to secure cannulae with a semipermeable film dressing rather than bandage. Nothing replaces careful observation of these sites by the nurse, as even intravenous delivery pumps are not considered reliable in detecting extravasation (Phelps and Helms 1993). Management of the resulting injury is essential as extensive tissue death could result in further damage with disastrous consequences.

The commonest method of management is the use of a sterile polythene bag containing a hydrogel (Thomas *et al.* 1987) or hydrogel covered with film. In extreme cases debridement, grafting and secondary reconstruction may be necessary (Yosowitz *et al.* 1975). Nurses must measure and document the position of the injury, the amount and type of wound tissue (e.g. necrotic, sloughy or granulating) and the extent and spread of erythema.

Nursing model for Samantha

When dealing with such a young infant the nurse's role will depend largely on interaction with Samantha's parents, but the type of nursing care given to Samantha's wound could have a profound effect on the rest of her life. The damage has been done, but further deterioration of the wound could result in her losing the use of her foot, or even the foot itself.

When choosing a model for Samantha consider the following priorities of care:

- the *trauma* to the parents having their new baby become so ill in a short space of time
- their *understanding* of the situation: do they know what has caused the injury to Samantha's foot?
- do they realize the potential problems that could arise from *mismanagement* of the wound?
- Samantha still has to *recover* fully from her septicaemia
- Samantha is experiencing *pain* when her foot is handled; this may discourage her parents from picking her up and cuddling her
- do the nurses understand the *legal* implications of this baby's care?

Look at the emphasized points: *trauma, understanding, mismanagement, recover, pain* and *legal.* All these points focus on the parents', nurses' and baby's

Table 4.1   *Use of the FANCAP mnemonic to plan Samantha's care*

	Physiological	Psychological	Sociological
Fluids	Needs to maintain necessary fluid intake orally and intravenously	Parents may not wish further IV fluids to be given because of extravasation	
Aeration	Necrotic tissue to be removed to facilitate healing of wound	Parents need to understand *how* and *why* necrotic tissue is removed	
Nutrition	Needs bottle feeds to be introduced	Parents frightened to feed baby owing to illness	Mother unsure how to feed baby
Communication	Doctors and nurses need to explain implications of injury Documentation essential	Parents frightened or angry at hospital, doctors and nurses as to why this injury has occurred	Parents may consider legal action against hospital
Activity	Baby needs to be cuddled and handled normally Left foot needs to regain normal movement		Parents need to understand importance of bonding
Pain	Dressings chosen that minimize pain on removal Do not restrict movement of foot	Nurses and parents frightened to change dressings if causing Samantha distress and pain	

perceptions of the situation. The type of environment that the baby is nursed in will greatly affect the parents' perception of this situation. An environment full of equipment and staff busying themselves with the baby may alienate the parents, and they will feel they are not being told everything. Although in Samantha's case her physiological care is important, the nurse must concentrate also on the psychological and sociological parameters to help the parents deal with their baby's illness. Riehl's interaction model addresses these issues (Riehl 1980), and she advocates the use of the FANCAP system (Fluids, Aeration, Nutrition, Communication, Activity and Pain) developed by Abbey (1980) to assess patients' needs. This can be applied to Samantha's needs as shown in Table 4.1.

Practice points

- Some of the problems have been highlighted; can you identify any others?
- The management of the wound can be achieved with the use of a hydrogel as previously outlined, which can be covered by either using a sterile plastic bag or using film dressings. The bag method is preferable because the wounds are visible, and pain is minimized as there is no trauma when removal takes place, as might occur with overzealous use of films.
- The management of this situation should be organized by an experienced paediatric team leader as it is essential that parents and nurses are kept informed of the implications of this type of injury.

Histiocytosis X

Histiocytosis X is a rare congenital disorder. The case described in Case Study 4.2 illustrates the problems of managing perineal wounds in babies.

Case Study 4.2
Histiocytosis

Simon James had been a healthy, normal baby until he was 5 months old, when he developed a generalized rash. This was initially diagnosed as eczema and treated by his general practitioner with emollients and steroid creams, both of which had little effect.

He was referred to a dermatologist, who admitted him to hospital for further investigation and treatment. Skin biopsies of the rash revealed a diagnosis of Langerhans' cell histiocytosis X. Within 5 days of admission Simon's condition deteriorated and he required artificial ventilation owing to respiratory distress. In conjunction with his general deterioration, Simon's rash had broken down and ulcerated, with large areas of necrotic eschar covering his abdomen and perineum (Figure 4.2). The perineal area was also contaminated with urine and faeces, and the staff of the paediatric intensive care unit were having trouble keeping a dressing on such a small infant.

Simon's mother was a single parent and lived in poor social circumstances. She had limited understanding of the severity of her son's condition and found it distressing to see his wound dressings being changed, as often they would stick to the skin causing Simon to cry.

Aetiology

Congenital abnormalities

Anatomical defects present at birth are classified as congenital abnormalities. This includes, but is not limited to, hereditary disorders.

Congenital abnormalities occur for several reasons. They can be inherited, caused by an embryological defect or can be idiopathic. About 1 in 100 babies is born with a severe malformation, accounting for 1 in 5 stillbirths and 1 in 10 infant deaths.

Histiocytosis X

Histiocytosis X is an extremely rare disorder that affects mainly children under the age of 2 years. The disorder derives its name from the type of body cell involved, the histiocyte (macrophage), with -*osis* meaning increased numbers, and X denoting that the cause is unknown. There are two main types of histiocytosis X, single system and multisystem. In single-system histiocytosis X only one organ in the body is affected, whereas in multi-system disease more than one organ is involved. This disorder is often confused with malignant disease; histiocytosis X is not a type of cancer. The histiocytes do not multiply in situ in an unorganized way, but tend to migrate to a site in abnormal numbers or stray outside their normal tissue compartment. Children with histiocytosis X have a deficiency of a certain type of white blood cell, the suppressor lymphocyte (Riggs and Bale 1993).

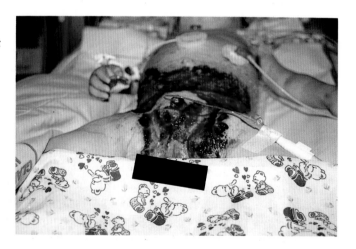

Figure 4.2 *Simon James with a large necrotic area on the groin and abdomen.*

Figure 4.3 *Simon following wound debridement with hydrogel and hydrocellular dressings. The dressings have been held in place with his napkin.*

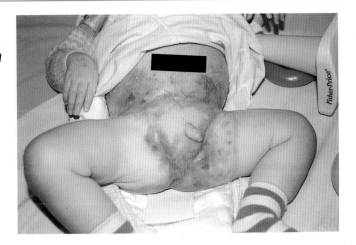

Prognosis varies. A high incidence of spontaneous remission occurs in single-system disease. Although patients with multisystem disease may spontaneously remit, these children often need treatment. Generally, the younger the child when diagnosed and the more organs involved, the poorer the prognosis. When histiocytosis is diagnosed in older children the disease often runs a more chronic course and may not be life-threatening, although there is associated morbidity leaving the child with chronic problems.

Management

Managing a wound in the perineum is a difficult nursing problem. Faecal and urinary contamination in a young infant with no bladder or bowel control is inevitable. Frequent wound hygiene is required to keep the bacterial count as low as possible, in combination with dressings that are easily and quickly changed. Use of a hydrogel together with a hydrocellular dressing may seem an expensive option, but several points need to be considered:

i)   Pain and distress are avoided using these dressings
ii) Hydrogels are quickly and easily removed when changing a napkin
iii) The treatment is effective (Figure 4.3)

Nursing model for Simon

Simon was a previously well infant; both he and his mother now have to *adapt* to the changes in his health status. A model that deals with *loss* of adaptation to ill-health is Roy's adaptation model (Roy 1980), which can be used to plan Simon's care as shown in Tables 4.2 and 4.3.

Table 4.2 Use of Roy's adaptation model to assess Simon's care

Life area	Assessment Level I — Behaviour	Assessment Level 2 — Stimuli		
		Focal	Contextual	Residual
Physiological				
nutrition	Not taking food orally	Unconscious	Mechanical ventilation	
elimination	No bladder or bowel control	Not yet learnt	Physiological development	
oxygenation	Unable to breathe spontaneously	Disease process		
regulation	Necrotic wound areas over perineum and abdomen	Disease process		Rash previously undiagnosed
	Dressings not staying in place	Difficult area to dress	Inexperience of staff dealing with wound	
	Wound contamination	Bladder and bowel incontinence	No continence aids in use	
	Infection of wounds	Cross-contamination from staff Immunosuppressed by disease	High-risk hospital area	
Rest and exercise	Normal activity stopped Nursed in frightening environment	Sudden onset of illness	Intensive therapy unit setting	
Self-concept	No familiar surroundings to lessen anxiety		Hospital surroundings	Never been in hospital
	Mother unable to understand severity of condition	Sudden onset of illness	Lack of intellectual skills	
Role function	Mother unable to provide care, loss of mother role	Mother excluded from care	Lack of social skills to cope	
Interdependency	Dependent on staff to provide care	Child too ill, needs specialist staff		No previous experience in hospital
	Mother feels helpless		No support from family, single mother	No previous experience in hospital
	Mother distressed at dressing changes	Not always present when dressings done	Lack of understanding of dressing procedure	No previous hospital experience

Table 4.3   *Care plan for Simon*

Problem	Goal	Intervention
Unable to breathe spontaneously (A)	Restore oxygenation to normal level	Artificial ventilation
Lack of nutrition (A)	Provide normal nutrition	IV nutrition (check)
Wound contamination from urine (A)	Prevention of urinary incontinence soiling wound	Indwelling catheterization until wound healed
Large amount of necrotic tissue over perineum and abdomen (A)	Removal of necrotic tissue to facilitate healing	Daily application of hydrogel to promote autolysis
Contamination of wound with faeces (A)	Removal of faeces from wound site	Highly absorbent hydrocellular dressing (Allevyn) to remove excess faecal fluid from wound site
Dressings not staying in place	Minimize disturbance of dressing	Secure with baby's nappy over Allevyn sheet
Wound infection (P)	Prevent introduction of infection	Strict asepsis when dressing wound Hand-washing between contacts and when handling soiled napkins
Lack of normal environment (A)	Minimize fear of environment	Staff always to talk, touch and smile with baby Avoid excess use of alarm systems on machines Keep familiar toys and pictures around bed area
Loss of role for mother	Promote mother's involvement	Include mother in care where possible Explain to her why particular treatments are carried out Encourage her to talk to and touch baby
Mother unable to understand severity of condition	Explain in clear terms child's prognosis	Doctors and nurses to use non-medical terms to explain condition Inform mother of changes Do not talk 'over' mother, always with her Involve social worker/health visitor to assess home conditions
Mother anxious at surroundings	Minimize her anxiety level	Encourage mother to voice fears to staff Allow time alone with baby if requested Allow time for her to ask questions
Mother distressed at dressing changes	Ensure pain-free dressing changes	Change dressings daily Soak dressings off if signs of adherence Allow mother to help if desired Explain nature and action of dressing products

(A), actual problem; (P), potential problem.

Practice points

- The emphasis of this care plan is placed on minimizing the trauma of being nursed in a 'high technology' area.
- The mother should be involved in Simon's care, but only when and if she desires it.
- Her distress at the dressing changes is possibly the way in which she expresses her general anxiety about his overall condition. However, it is one area of care in which she could be involved, provided she has adequate support and guidance.

Infectious Diseases

One of the most serious infectious diseases in small children is meningitis, as described in Case Study 4.3.

Case Study 4.3
Infectious diseases

Lisa Evans, a previously healthy 11–month–old girl, has been ill for the past week with a cold, cough and sore throat.

Her condition deteriorated one evening when she became very hot and began to vomit. Following three episodes of vomiting she became listless and appeared to be losing consciousness. Her mother called the general practitioner who arranged her immediate admission to hospital with suspected meningococcal meningitis.

Following admission Lisa was transferred to the intensive care unit for intubation and intravenous antibiotic therapy. By the following day she had developed a purpuric rash over her trunk, buttocks and legs and she was diagnosed as having meningococcal septicaemia (Figure 4.4).

Within the next 3 days the purpuric rash had spread to involve both arms and was blistering, necrotic and wet. Lisa had responded well to her antibiotics and was breathing spontaneously, but remained nursed in a high-dependency area off the intensive care unit.

Epidemiology

Despite the numerous medical advances that have taken place in paediatrics, the mortality and morbidity rates from meningitis have not decreased. Almost 10% of affected children die and permanent defects affect over 30% of the survivors (Levin and Heyderman 1991). The incidence of

Figure 4.4 *Purpuric rash of meningococcal meningitis in a 7 year old child.*

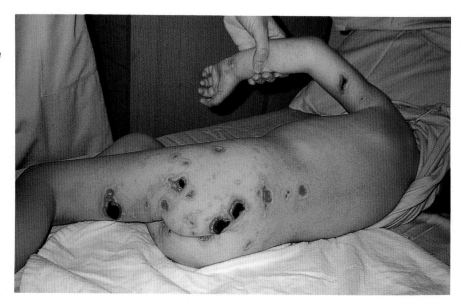

Table 4.4 *Incidence of bacterial meningitis*

Age group	Rate per 1000 population
Neonate	232
1 month–11 months	65
1 year–4 years	16

From Levin and Heyderman (1991)

bacterial meningitis is highest in the first 12 months following birth, with the rates falling as childhood progresses (Table 4.4).

Aetiology

The incidence within industrialized countries, far from falling, is increasing (Kaplan 1989). Organisms causing meningitis vary; interestingly, different pathogens affect specific age groups:

- neonate — group B streptococci, coliform bacteria
- 1 month onwards — *Haemophilus influenzae, Neisseria meningitidis, Streptococcus pneumoniae*
- 1–4 years — *Haemophilus influenzae*

Diagnosis of meningitis is difficult, with symptoms being vague and in the first instance identical to many other, less dangerous, childhood illnesses. Typically the infant will develop a generalized febrile illness which can rapidly worsen and the infant's condition deteriorates. The purpuric rash of meningococcal meningitis is associated with an overwhelming infection with gram-negative diplococcus or meningococcus, thus causing haemorrhage through toxic damage to the capillaries. Skin damage from this rash can often be so severe that full-thickness skin loss and ulceration result in permanent damage (Lester 1992).

Diagnosis is based on

i)   The presence of a non-specific febrile illness
ii) Raised intracranial pressure, clinical signs of which include reduced and declining level of consciousness, extensor hypertonia, cranial nerve palsy, dilated pupils, bradycardia and high blood pressure
iii) Positive blood culture
iv) Lumbar puncture to obtain cerebrospinal fluid, which will detect raised levels of white cells and protein and reduced glucose concentration

Management

Patient outcome is dependent on early diagnosis and treatment. Third-generation cephalosporins offer a safer and more effective alternative to the previously popular antibiotic regimens of chloramphenicol and penicillins. These infants can best be nursed on paediatric intensive care units with aggressive support of cardiovascular function, elective ventilation and measures to reduce raised intracranial pressure. If the infant survives this acute stage of the illness, bacterial toxins can cause other problems such as vascular damage. Ulceration can be treated with excision and grafting, a process that will hasten healing but will depend on the child's general condition and the availability of plastic surgery. Alternatively, hydrogels, hydrocolloids or silver sulphadiazine creams will soften eschar and deslough the wounds (Lester 1992). This may be the easiest option for parent and child for care that continues in the community. All these materials are readily available on prescription at home. Hydrocolloid sheets are occlusive and permit bathing and playing, without risking wound contamination from the outside environment. At this age babies are crawling, rolling and learning to stand; they may also pull at dressings that are not firmly fixed. Difficulty may arise with the use of hydrocolloids as the dressing stays in place for several days at a time, so wound inspection would not be possible on a daily basis. Hydrogels and silver sulphadiazine may need to be used in conjunction with a film dressing to make this a practical option. Again, bathing, playing and crawling around would not disturb the dressings. Frequent wound inspection would be possible as the dressing would need to be changed on a daily basis.

Nursing model for Lisa

Lisa's condition is life-threatening, and although the nurse needs to establish a good relationship with her parents her first priority will be assessing Lisa's physical condition.

The correct management of the child's wound at this stage may avoid or minimize the scarring that could result from her meningococcal rash. Using Peplau's model, assess Lisa's needs under the SOAP structure (Peplau 1952):

S — Subjective feelings and experiences of the patient or parent, e.g. mother concerned at the large amount of 'black scabs' on wound

O — Objective observation by nurse, e.g. large areas of necrotic tissue preventing wound from healing

A — Formal assessment and identification of problem. Problem statement or goal: necrotic tissue requiring removal

P — Plan of action:
　　　apply hydrogel to facilitate autolysis
　　　apply low-adherent dressings

S — Mother anxious that Lisa will not recover from meningitis

O — Vital signs now within normal limits and baby recovering:
　　　baby breathing spontaneously
　　　displays no signs of cerebral irritation

A — Mother's anxiety level high

P — Provide mother with information and reassurance of baby's recovery:
　　　allow mother to stay with baby
　　　inform mother of changes in baby's condition
　　　allow mother to participate in baby's care

Figure 4.5 *Baby Lisa showing wounds healed.*

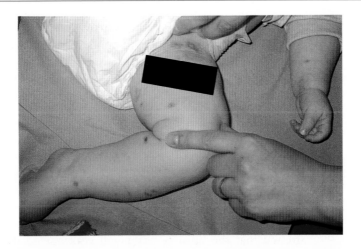

- Observations could also be made concerned with recording the wound size, ensuring wounds do not become macerated and that removal of the dressings is painless for the baby.
- The mother will need counselling regarding the length of time treatment of her baby's wounds may take and how she can help care for Lisa during this period (Figure 4.5).

Thermal Injuries

Wounds from burns and scalds in young children are frequently found in nursing practice. An example of an accidental injury of this type is given in Case Study 4.4.

Case Study 4.4 Thermal injuries

Lucy Llewellyn is just 2 years old and was admitted to Primrose Ward at 10 a.m. as an emergency. Lucy, the youngest of three children, had gone into the kitchen unsupervised this morning and reached up to the kitchen unit to get her teddy bear. Unfortunately she had not seen the full cup of tea her father had left just on the edge and tipped it over herself, scalding her shoulder, upper arm and chest. Her mother, alerted by Lucy's screams, had the foresight to immediately remove the clothing and run the scalded areas under the tap for 10 minutes, and cover the area with a clean tea-towel. The father called an ambulance which took her to the local hospital where Lucy was treated for a deep, partial-thickness injury to her shoulder and upper arm, and a superficial partial-thickness injury to her chest. Although these injuries were serious, the mother's quick action had prevented further damage.

Epidemiology

Thermal injuries from flame, burns and scalds are extremely common injuries for young children. Around 2500–3000 children are admitted to hospital as a result of scald injuries, with as many children again admitted with burns in England and Wales (Forshaw 1991). In the 1–5 year age group, scalding is due mostly to hot drinks, teapots, saucepans and baths (Lawrence 1987a).

Management

Correct and prompt first-aid management of burns and scalds can reduce the depth of tissue damage substantially. Immediate application of cold water to the scald rapidly quenches residual heat and eases pain (Lawrence 1987b). Parents, however, may be distressed at their screaming child, not know how long to apply cold water, and be alarmed by seeing skin peel off. It should be stressed that the burn or scald will continue to develop with redness and blistering and appear to enlarge. Seconds are often lost by removal of clothing, which should also be drenched to save time (Petch 1993).

Thermal injuries are classified according to depth (Centre for Medical Education 1992):

- *Partial-thickness skin loss* — fluid lost from the burn wound either forms blisters under damaged skin or exudate from areas where the outer layers have been lost.
  i) Superficial partial-thickness skin loss — the epidermis and superficial layers of the dermis are destroyed. Hair follicles, sebaceous and sweat glands are, however, spared. From these epithelial structures migration of cells rapidly occurs to provide an intact surface within 10–14 days. This type of burn is painful as the nerve endings of the dermis have not been damaged. The wound usually heals without scarring.
  ii) Deep partial-thickness skin loss — a greater part of the dermis is lost, and little of the skin appendages remain. Healing is delayed. Sensation is altered — patient has blunting of pin-prick sensation.
- *Full-thickness skin loss* — there are no surviving epithelial elements in full-thickness loss. The burn can only heal by contraction and by migration of existing epithelial cells at the edges of the wound. The wound may look pale and charred, and coagulated veins may be visible. No sensation is present on testing.

Nursing the child following injury

On admission to the children's ward an initial assessment of the child will take into account that the child has not been prepared for admission and may be very frightened. As a result the child may be fractious and crying, frightened and clinging to her parents. On admission the nurse will aim to:

i)   Use a calm and friendly approach to the child and family to comfort and reassure the child. The child will be assured that her mother or father will be able to stay with her so that she will not be left alone.

ii)   Encourage the parents to cuddle and care for the child. Intravenous infusions and other equipment need not prevent parents from maintaining close contact with their child.

iii)   Explain to the child and parents, using terms they will understand, any procedures that may need to be performed.

iv)   Be non-judgemental, to reassure the parents that blame is not being apportioned. Some parents may want to talk about the accident, and may be obviously distressed. The nurse aims to restore the parents' confidence and self-esteem as they may be feeling inadequate and guilty.

Longer-term aims of nursing care are:

i)   To help the parents understand that their child may take time in adapting to the new environment and that behavioural disturbances are to be expected. Their child may become aggressive and difficult or, alternatively, may become quiet and withdrawn. Behavioural regression may take many forms and parents need the reassurance that this is temporary.

ii)   To encourage the child to become independent again, and restore her self-confidence.

iii)   To introduce the child to play leaders, nursery nurses and teachers, where appropriate, to minimize boredom. In addition, televisions, videos and computer games can help to alleviate boredom.

Over a period of time the nurse may be able to take on a health educator role in helping the parents to understand how the accident happened and how it may be prevented in the future. Gaffin suggested how nurses may achieve this in a way which does not simply tell the parents how the accident happened (Gaffin 1991). This involves looking at a number of factors contributing to the accident and including the child, the agent involved (e.g. the cup of tea), and the physical and social context in which the accident happened.

Non-accidental injury

In the accident and emergency department parents are likely to be closely questioned on how the accident happened, and what action they took subsequently. The child may also be asked what happened — although in Lucy's case this would not be admissible as she is shocked and distressed. Staff will always ascertain whether the distribution of injury fits the history given by the parents.

Effects of hypertrophic scarring

Unfortunately the hypertrophic scarring following a burn or scald can be a constant disfiguring reminder to the child of the causative accident. Hypertrophic scars are red, firm and thickened and cause intensive itching (see Chapter 1).

Although hypertrophic scarring usually flattens as the scar matures, there is evidence that the use of constant, long-term pressure can prevent its formation (Carr-Collins 1992). Specially made elastic garments can be used to apply pressure on the torso and limbs and help realignment of the collagen fibres. These are worn for 24 hours daily and removed only for cleansing or bathing for the first 9 months (Pape 1993) for a period of up to 2 years. Garments will need frequent replacement in the growing child and great care is required to ensure they are comfortable and well-fitting. The wearing of such garments can have a profound effect on small children and will affect all sorts of normal activities of a 2-year-old, such as swimming and the wearing of dresses.

Success has also been achieved with topical application of silicone gel sheeting, although its mode of action is unclear. The sheeting is cut to size and secured with adhesive tape, and needs to be worn for several weeks day and night (Perkins *et al.* 1983). Perhaps a more acceptable alternative for children, silicone gel sheeting is expensive and its availability limited to specialist centres.

Treatment of burns and scalds

On admission to an accident and emergency department a thorough history of the accident will be taken from the parents and/or child.

For major burn injuries or deep skin loss around the face and neck the main concern is maintenance of a clear airway. Estimation of the percentage size of the burn is calculated using the Lund and Browder chart (Figure 4.6). The child's weight is taken and assessment of fluid requirements calculated. If the burn is over 10% of the body surface pain relief and tetanus toxoid will be given where required, depending on the depth and type of burn injury.

Wound dressings

The burn or scald should be swabbed prior to cleansing, to ascertain the type of bacteria present in the wound. Bacterial colonization of all thermal wounds occurs following injury but generally causes no problems with healing (Ayliffe *et al.* 1993). Certain organisms, however, may cause particular problems, especially *Staphylococcus aureus* which can result in toxic shock syndrome.

Cleansing should be performed with saline (see Chapter 2) using irrigation techniques. Dead epithelium and blisters are removed using sterile

Figure 4.6 *Lund and Browder chart (with kind permission of Smith & Nephew Pharmaceuticals).*

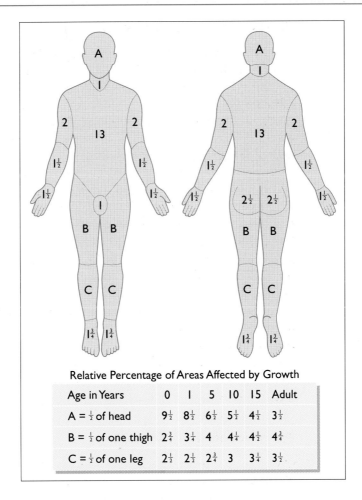

Relative Percentage of Areas Affected by Growth

Age in Years	0	1	5	10	15	Adult
A = $\frac{1}{2}$ of head	$9\frac{1}{2}$	$8\frac{1}{2}$	$6\frac{1}{2}$	$5\frac{1}{2}$	$4\frac{1}{2}$	$3\frac{1}{2}$
B = $\frac{1}{2}$ of one thigh	$2\frac{3}{4}$	$3\frac{1}{4}$	4	$4\frac{1}{4}$	$4\frac{1}{2}$	$4\frac{3}{4}$
C = $\frac{1}{2}$ of one leg	$2\frac{1}{2}$	$2\frac{1}{2}$	$2\frac{3}{4}$	3	$3\frac{1}{4}$	$3\frac{1}{2}$

scissors, with debridement of necrotic material under strict aseptic conditions. Deep dermal burns will require surgical debridement in theatre followed by excision and grafting.

Following cleansing, burns should be covered with a low-adherent dressing.

Films and hydrocolloids (Forshaw 1993) will provide moist wound healing and protection to the wounds. Superficial burns with low exudate can be covered with low-adherent woven gauzes. Deeper wounds with large amounts of exudate or infection can be dressed with alginates. Silver sulphadiazine (Flamazine) is widely used as a prophylactic agent, particularly against *Pseudomonas aeruginosa* infection and is useful on hands (in plastic bags), ears and genital areas (Wound Healing Research Unit 1994).

Nursing model for Lucy

There are many issues at stake for Lucy and her family. The nurse on the ward needs to build a strong, trusting relationship with the toddler and her parents. As with Samantha (Case Study 4.1), it is important to look at psychological and sociological aspects, as well as physiological care for Lucy and her parents. Riehl's model is therefore a useful framework for the initial assessment. Look at the problems identified below and consider how you can help child and parents. Look at it from the parents' and child's points of view, i.e. their definition of the situation.

- *Physiological* (A, actual; P, potential):
    pain due to burn injury (A)
    risk of infection in wound site (P)
    hypertrophic scarring following wound healing (P)
    dressings adhering to wound causing painful dressing change (P)
    child not wanting nurses to change the dressings (P)
- *Psychological*:
    parents, particularly father, feeling guilty about accident (A)
    child not understanding what has happened to her (A)
    repeated questioning in accident and emergency department and ward reinforcing feelings of guilt (P)
- *Sociological*:
    child suddenly put in unfamiliar surroundings owing to emergency admission (A)
    lack of parental knowledge with regard to prevention of further accidents (A)
    parents separated from other children (A)
    parents labelled by ward staff as uncaring and careless (P)
    child at risk of non-accidental injury (A)

Practice points

- There are many psychological factors influencing the parents, but the child may have psychological effects long-term, so this should be considered now.
- This case highlights the need for the specialist skills of trained paediatric nurses when dealing with traumatic injuries in infants. How the care is planned will depend on the experience of the nurse. Inexperienced practitioners may not even identify some of these problems and may not be equipped to provide the required management.
- Think of the specific skills that a nurse requires to deal with this case.

Animal Bite Wounds

Facial wounds in children are commonly caused by bites from animals (usually dogs). Look at the example in Case Study 4.5.

Case Study 4.5
Injury from dog bite

Sister Mathews is the practice nurse working in a general practice surgery serving a counsil estate in a large city. One morning Sally Arnold, a child 8 years old was brought in screaming and hysterical by her mother, with her face covered in blood. When the nurse had calmed both mother and child she elicited that the child had been playing with their pet mongrel dog who had suddenly jumped up and bitten her cheek.

Sister Mathews irrigated the wound with copious amounts of saline and examined the size and shape of the affected area. Sally had sustained a single laceration above her left cheekbone which measured 1.3 cm in breadth and 0.5 cm in depth. The initial treatment was closure of the wound with sterile adhesive strips while waiting for the doctor to examine the child.

The doctor, who had only had limited experience with suturing facial wounds, arranged for mother and child to go to the city hospital's accident and emergency department. A plastic surgeon examined the wound and, having excluded damage to the underlying tissues, the wound edges were carefully brought together using paper skin closure strips. The child was prescribed a course of penicillin elixir and asked to return to the hospital in 7 days.

Aetiology

Animal bites are a common cause of facial injury. In most Western countries 90% are caused by dog bites (Wishan and Huang 1989) and 50–75% affect children (Boenning *et al.* 1983). In children facial wounds are involved in 80% of such injuries (Lackmann *et al.* 1992). As an added hazard animal bites carry the risk of diseases such as tetanus and rabies, although these are less common than infections caused by micro-organisms of the normal flora of the animal's mouth and throat.

Management

Bites are best treated within the first 12–24 hours. Prophylactic broad-spectrum antibiotics are advised in high-risk patients. Skin closure is best achieved using adhesive strips and fine biocompatible sutures (Al-Khaleeb 1995). Where sutures are used, early removal is recommended to help prevent scarring. In facial injuries a plastic surgeon is often consulted prior to attempting suturing to ensure that the best cosmetic effect is obtained. Areas that warrant special attention include:

i)   The lip — repair of lip lacerations needs to be performed with respect to the vermilion border so that puckering is prevented

ii) The eyelids — repair of injuries to the area surrounding the eye can take place only after the ophthalmologist has examined the eye

iii) Haematomas need to be carefully evacuated prior to wound closure

iv)   Damage to bone, ducts, blood vessels and nerves should be repaired prior to wound closure

v)   Extensive tissue loss — depending on the site and extent of the injury, free grafts, pedicle grafts, flaps and tissue expansion can be used

For at least the first 3 months following facial injury the parents are advised to avoid exposure of the child's face to direct sunlight and prolonged soaking of the skin in water.

Nursing model of care for Sally

Before assessing this child's need, look at the previous section. Can you answer the following questions?

- Why was it necessary to irrigate the wound with copious amounts of saline?
- What other information should the Sister obtain about the circumstances of the accident?
- What course of action should the nurse take with regard to the dog?
- Why was the doctor reluctant to suture the wound?
- Why did the child require other management, e.g. antibiotics and/or tetanus vaccine?

Practice points

- You should be able to answer the above questions and include them in your plan of care. If you cannot answer, re-read the previous chapter on management of traumatic wounds.
- Once you have obtained the relevant information, what type of model could you use? See if you can write out a detailed plan including all the management issues raised.

Summary

This chapter has dealt mainly with wounds that have a traumatic aetiology — the most common type of wound that nurses have to treat. In this age group it can be seen that direct management of the traumatic wound can often appear straightforward.

Difficulties arise with the psychological and sociological traumas surrounding wound care in babies and infants. The models that have been chosen to assess the care in each of the case studies have largely concentrated on these important areas, and are not easy options on busy paediatric units. They do, hopefully, encourage the practitioner to think about such issues as:

- communication skills — with child, parents and team members
- legal and moral aspects of care — documentation, non-disclosure of information, choice of treatments
- organizational skills — planned management of care
- dressing choices — alleviation of painful dressing changes, minimization of scarring

Further Reading

Lawrence JC, Kidson A & Lilly HA (1992) An adherent semipermeable film dressing for burns. *Journal of Wound Care* 1(2): 10–11.

Partridge J (1993) The psychological effects of facial disfigurement. *Journal of Wound Care* 2(3): 168–171.

Forshaw A (1987) After care for the burned child and his family: do they need it? *Burns* 13: 522–524.

Lawrence JC & Cason C (1994) Kettle scalds. *Journal of Wound Care* 3(6): 289–292.

Douglas J (1993) *Psychology and Nursing Children*. London: Macmillan.

Craft MJ & Denely JA (1990) *Nursing Interventions for Infants and Children*. Philadelphia: WB Saunders.

White A (1991) Caring for children. Towards partnership with families. London: Edward Arnold.

Müller DJ, Harris PJ, Wattley L & Taylor JD (1992) Nursing children, psychology, research and practice, 2nd edn. London: Chapman & Hall.

Brunner LS & Suddarth DS, adapted by Weller BF (1986) Lippincott manual of paediatric nursing, 2nd edn. London: Harper & Row.

References

Abbey J (1980) The FANCAP assessment scheme. In: Riehl JP & Roy C (eds) *Conceptual Models for Nursing Practice*. New York: Appleton-Century-Crofts.

Al-Khaleeb T & Shepherd JP (1995) The management and repair of wounds of the face. *Journal of Wound Care*, 4(8): 359–362.

Ayliffe GAF, Lowbury EJF, Geddes AM & Williams JD (1993) *Control of Hospital Infection — A Practical Handbook*, 3rd edn. London: Chapman & Hall.

Boenning DA, Fleisher GR & Campos JM (1983) Dog bites in children: epidemiology, microbiology and penicillin prophylactic therapy. *American Journal of Emergency Medicine* 88: 17–21.

Bryne WJ (1990) The gastrointestinal tract. In: Bekerman RE & Eleigram R (eds) *Essentials of Paediatrics*. Philadelphia: Saunders.

Carr-Collins JA (1992) Pressure techniques for the prevention of hypertrophic scar. *Clinical Plastic Surgery* 19(3): 733–743.

Centre for Medical Education (1992) *The Wound Programme*. University of Dundee.

Forshaw A (1993) Hydrocolloid dressings in paediatric wound care. *Journal of Wound Care*, 2(4): 209.

Gaffin J (1991) The role of the nurse in accident prevention. In: Mead D & Sibert J (eds) *The Injured Child*. London: Scutari Press.

Kaplan SL (1989) *Recent Advances in Bacterial Meningitis*. London: Academic Press.

Lackmann GM, Draf W, Isselstein G & Tollner U (1992) Surgical treatment of facial dog bite injuries in children. *Journal of Craniomaxillofacial Surgery* 20: 81–86.

Lawrence JC (1987a) Burns to children. *Medical Research Council News* 36: 25–36.

Lawrence JC (1987b) British Burn Association recommended first aid for burns and scalds. *Burns* 13(2): 153.

Lester R (1992) Wound problems with meningococcal septicaemia. *Journal of Wound Care* 1(2): 24–25.

Levin M & Heyderman RS (1991) Bacterial meningitis. In: David TS (ed.) *Paediatrics*. Edinburgh: Churchill Livingstone.

Llewellyn N (1994) Pain assessment and the use of morphine. *Paediatric Nursing* 6(1): 25–30.

McCaffery M & Beebe A (1989) *Pain Clinical Manual for Nursing Practice*. St Louis: Mosby.

Mead D (1991) Nursing management of the injured child in the ward. In: Mead D & Sibert J (eds) *The Injured Child*. London: Scutari Press.

Melforth N (1995) Strategies to reduce children's perception of pain. *Nursing Times* 91(2): 34–35.

Pape SA (1993) The management of scars. *Journal of Wound Care* 2(6): 354–360.

Peplau H (1952) *Interpersonal Relations in Nursing*. New York: GP Putman.

Perkins K, Davey RB, Wallis KA (1983) Silicone gel: a new treatment for burn scars and contractures. *Burns* 9(3): 201–204.

Petch N & Cason CG (1993) Examining first aid received by burn and scald patients. *Journal of Wound Care* 2(2): 102–105.

Phelps SJ & Helms RA (1983) Risk factors affecting infiltrations of peripheral venous lines in infants. *Journal of Pediatrics* 111(3): 384–389.

RCN (1992) *Paediatric Nursing: A Philosophy of Care*. Issues in Nursing and Health. London: RCN.

Riehl JP (1980) The Riehl interaction model. In: Riehl JP & Roy C (eds) *Conceptual Models for Nursing Practice*. New York: Appleton-Century-Crofts.

Riggs RL & Bale S (1993) Management of necrotic wounds as a complication of histiocytosis X. *Journal of Wound Care* 2(5): 260–261.

Roy C (1980) The Roy adaptation model. In: Riehl JP & Roy C (eds) *Conceptual Models for Nursing Practice*. Nw York: Appleton-Century-Crofts.

Thomas S, Rowe HN, Keats J & Morgan RJH (1987) A new approach to the management of extravasation injury in neonates. *Pharmaceutical Journal* 239 (6457): pp 584–585.

Tomlinson D (1987). To clean or not to clean? *Nursing Times* 83(9): 71–75.

Wishan PM & Huang A (1989) Pet-associated injuries: the trouble with children's best friend. *Children Today* 18: 24–27.

Wound Healing Research Unit (1994) *Wound Management — Good Practice Guidance*. NHS Cymru, Wales.

Yosowitz P, Eklan DA, Shaw RC & Parsons RW (1975) Peripheral intravenous infiltration necrosis. *Annals of Surgery* 182(5): 553–556.

Young T (1995) Wound healing in neonates. *Journal of Wound Care* 4(6): 285–288.

5

Wound Care in Teenagers

Key issues

This chapter outlines the most common wound problems encountered by the teenager.

Clinical Case Studies

Aetiology and management of:

- A young boy sustaining chemical burns caused by battery acid
- Pressure sore in a young girl with spina bifida
- Traumatic injuries due to a road traffic accident

Nursing Models

Examples of their application to practice are taken from:

- Roper's activities of living model
- Orem's model
- Roy's adaptation model

Practice Points

As you read through this chapter concentrate on the following:

- Inadequate wound management which may affect the rest of the teenager's life
- Aspects of privacy, body image and personal identity important to a teenager
- Emotional effects that injury may have on the teenager
- Devastating effect of disablement or disfigurement on the rest of the teenager's life

Introduction

Of all the phases of the life-cycle, adolescence is undoubtedly one of the most difficult. During the adolescent period the individual changes from a child into an adult and strives to achieve social and emotional maturity. Adolescents are prone to experimenting with all aspects of their life. This is likely to include alcohol, cigarettes and maybe drugs. Peer group pressure is strong. Being accepted by peers is a fundamental issue for youths. At this age individuals may set out to impress others by acting irresponsibly and taking unnecessary risks. The duration of adolescence and the age at which it occurs is difficult to determine, as each individual varies. Adolescence has been defined as being a phase of 'intellectual, social, emotional and physical change through which an individual progresses in passing from childhood to maturity' (British Paediatric Association 1989).

Common behavioural traits exhibited by adolescents include mood swings, rebellion, paranoia, self-preoccupation and antagonism. Coming to terms with the adult world can be an extremely traumatic time for the young individual. Illness and hospitalization of adolescents can be difficult when often their physical needs take precedence over their emotional needs. Health professionals, including nurses, seem to be less aware of the needs and rights of teenagers, especially when considering their independence, privacy and social needs (Gillies 1992). Very few adolescent wards are available in hospitals and teenagers tend to be placed either in paediatric wards or in adult wards. Wherever the teenager is cared for health professionals should try to accommodate their needs, which may include body image and personal identity issues, independence (social and financial) from parents, and help in communicating and developing social skills (Weller 1985).

Specific problems for adolescents being treated in hospital (Farrelly 1994) include:

- Lack of privacy
- Problems associated with change of body image
- Anxiety related to hospitalization
- Fear of rejection by their peer group
- Restriction of normal physical activities
- Fear of death in the seriously ill
- Loss of independence

The adolescent period is one in which accidental and traumatic injuries are common and both mortality and morbidity rates are high. Wounds frequently result from such injuries. In 1989 in the UK 3.5% of all male deaths and 2.2% of all female deaths were the result of accidents including violence (Central Statistical Office 1991).

Chemical Burns

Case Study 5.1 illustrates the case of a schoolboy injured in an industrial accident with corrosive materials.

Case Study 5.1 Chemical burns

David Oskim, a 17-year-old schoolboy, has always had a keen interest in cars and car maintenance. Last month he secured a Saturday job in the local garage as a trainee mechanic. He was particularly pleased as his father had just bought him a car and he was having driving lessons.

The garage owner was pleased to take David on because of his enthusiasm but also because he only needed to pay him a small amount of money. A hard-working, conscientious man, he had little time to give David a proper induction and assumed David was aware of the usual hazards of working in this environment.

One Saturday David was working on an engine which required him to remove and drain the battery. While lifting the battery out of its casing David let it slip and tipped battery acid over his forearm. The owner, who had not experienced this type of accident before, immediately led David to the washbasin, plunged his arm and hand in a basin of cold water and removed the sleeve of his overall. While telephoning for an ambulance he told David to keep his arm under the tap. On arrival at the accident and emergency department David was shocked and in a great deal of pain, having sustained a superficial partial-thickness burn to his forearm.

Aetiology

Industrial accidents are unfortunately still part of everyday working life. From a workforce of more than 800 000 in the West Midlands (Neale and Haine 1983) an average of 55 men per annum are seriously burnt (Lawrence 1990).

The level of first-aid these workers receive will greatly affect their prognosis and degree of injury. In Petch's study of first-aid received (Petch and Cason 1993) of the 18 patients admitted to the burns unit as a result of industrial accidents, only 7 had received satisfactory first-aid while 8 had received none at all (Table 5.1).

Table 5.1 *First aid received by a selection of patients admitted to the burns unit*

Patient group	First aid received		
	Satisfactory	Unsatisfactory	None
Children	15	3	6
Adults at home	9	3	10
Industrial cases	7	3	8
Other cases not in or around the home	2	3	2
Total	33	12	26

From Petch and Cason (1993)

Figure 5.1 *Chemical burn sustained following contact with cement.*

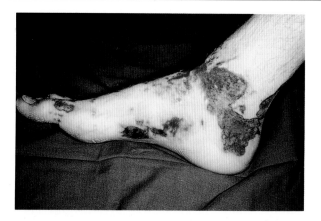

Management

The rapid removal of corrosive chemicals from the skin is an urgent first-aid requirement. Highly acid and alkaline substances are readily absorbed into the tissues causing rapid burning to the affected area (Figure 5.1). Irrigation of the burnt area with vast quantities of water should normally be commenced as soon as possible (but see below for exceptions). Any clothing in contact with the injured area should be cut away and the skin irrigation continued until an ambulance arrives or en route to the accident and emergency department. Full details of the nature and composition of the corrosive chemical causing the burn will be needed by the hospital, so every attempt should be made to identify the substance. Some chemicals have specific antidotes which can be given in the accident and emergency department. It is important to note that not all chemical burns should be irrigated with water. Substances containing metallic sodium, potassium and lithium should not be irrigated with water.

In hospital an assessment of the degree and extent of the burns will be made. The Lund and Browder chart (see Figure 4.7) is now considered to be a more effective method of assessing extent of burns injuries than the 'rule of nine' (Settle 1986). The depth of burn should be assessed and recorded. This can be done by estimating the loss of epidermis, dermis and appendages (see Chapter 4).

Treatment of small burns may be carried out in the accident and emergency department without the need for admitting the young person. Removal of dirt and devitalized tissue is essential. Where surgical debridement is needed to remove devitalized tissue, the hospital stay may be only a few days. The use of modern wound dressings for full-thickness burns is applicable where infection has been eliminated so that daily activity is relatively unaffected. Hydrogels, hydrocolloids, foams and alginates may all have a role to play.

- Hydrogels are comfortable, conformable, provide moisture at the wound bed, and can be used with semipermeable films, thus allowing bathing, etc.

- Hydrocolloids are occlusive, need infrequent dressing changes, comfortable and permit bathing
- Foams are comfortable and absorbent; some foams are adhesive
- Alginates are absorbent, comfortable, and can be used with pads or semipermeable films to allow bathing, etc.

Returning to normal activities, such as swimming and sports, may be facilitated by using occlusive dressings. Monitoring of the healing wound may be undertaken by the practice or district nurse in conjunction with the parents, though teenagers may wish to care for their own wounds on a day-to-day basis. Tetanus protection is essential for all types of burns, irrespective of depth. The choice of dressing material will depend on a thorough assessment of the patient, and especially the lifestyle of the adolescent will need to be taken into consideration.

The long-term consequences of a chemical burn may be disfiguring, with scarring of the affected area. The adolescent and parents may wish to take legal action against the employer if negligence is involved. The Health and Safety Act may be acted upon to prevent recurrence of such an accident, and procedures for handling chemicals may need to be reviewed.

Nursing model for David

Luckily for David his employer took the right course of first-aid action, although he should have ensured David had adequate Health and Safety advice before he took the job!

Table 5.2 *Assessment of David's problems (Case Study 5.1)*

Activities of living	Problem statements
Eliminating	Normal bowel action Urine output Cannot use right hand to attend to personal hygiene following elimination
Eating and drinking	Good diet and fluid intake but cannot eat very well with one hand
Working and playing	Unable to continue work, cannot write as right-handed. Future employment/education may be affected
Mobilizing	Just started driving lessons which he cannot continue
Sleeping	Arm and hand still quite painful, cannot get comfortable at night Worried about employment and school work
Personal cleansing	Cannot wash or shower very well
Expressing sexuality	Worried about effects of burns or scarring to his arm and hand

Although a partial-thickness burn should heal without scarring, the type of care David receives now may influence the rest of his life. Any injury to a hand, however superficial, should ideally be assessed by a plastic surgeon.

Use Roper's model (Roper *et al.* 1980) to assess David's care (Table 5.2).

The assessment reveals that David has the following major problems:

- Motor activities:
    cannot wash
    cannot eat normally
    cannot work
    cannot write
    cannot drive
    pain
- Psychosocial aspects:
    disruption in schooling
    anxiety
    self-image (effect of scarring)

Practice points

- For an apparently small injury there are many complications.
- The management of the burnt hand can best be achieved with silver sulpha-diazine in a sterile plastic bag; the arm can be covered with a film dressing or other low-adherent material. Neither arm nor hand will require grafting.
- Should there be any complications at a later date, documentation of treatment and wound assessment must be meticulous.
- Think about how this accident could have been avoided.

Pressure Sores

Pressure sores are normally associated with elderly patients, but can occur in young patients with disabilities such as spina bifida, discussed in Case Study 5.2.

Case Study 5.2
Pressure sores in a young, physically disabled teenager

Thirteen-year old Tracy Childs was born with spina bifida and has been paralysed from the waist down since birth. Incontinent of faeces and urine, Tracy has been hospitalized many times for urinary diversion and now has a permanent urostomy.

Tracy lives with her mother and father and younger brother John, who is 7 years old. The family house has been adapted for Tracy's wheelchair and has a downstairs bathroom with shower. Although dogged by episodes of ill-health, Tracy remains a cheerful and determined teenager who, with her devoted mother giving 24-hour-care, copes well with her disabilities.

Six weeks ago Tracy complained of feeling unwell and was diagnosed as having a urinary infection. Despite a course of oral antibiotics she became nauseated, confused and had a temperature of 40 °C. She was rushed into hospital where she received intravenous antibiotics and was, for several days, seriously ill. Unable to eat food, she lost 4.5 kg in weight and because of her position in bed and lack of her usual stoma bags urine leaked out around her conduit. This resulted on three occasions in Tracy lying in one position for several hours on wet sheets. When she finally became well she was put in an ordinary wheelchair without the pressure-relieving cushion which she would normally have in her wheelchair at home.

Tracy's mother was distressed at the apparent lack of attention to her daughter's needs. Although the staff were caring the ward was obviously inadequately staffed and lacked what Tracy's mother viewed as essential equipment. On her mother's insistence Tracy was discharged home as soon as her temperature became normal and prescribed an oral antibiotic regimen. The day after discharge, in the course of a blanket bath, Tracy's mother noticed two broken areas on the teenager's left hip and right ischial tuberosity. Two days later they became black in the middle and deep red around the outside. She was horrified, realizing these were pressure sores, and called the general practitioner, who sent the district nurse to assess the situation.

Aetiology

Spina bifida is caused by defective closure of the caudal neuropore towards the end of the fourth week of gestation. Spina bifida occulta (non-fusion of the spinal arches limited to vertebral defects) occurs in around 10% of the population. Although a small dimple or hair tuft can be seen, individuals are generally asymptomatic. However, spina bifida cystica is less common, occurring in 1 in 1000 births. The lesion is sac-like in appearance, with multiple unfused vertebrae. The lesions can be closed, with either the meninges alone (meningocele) or both the meninges and the spinal cord (meningomyelocele) within the sac. A more severe version, myeloschisis, occurs when an open neural tube is present without an overlying sac. Spina bifida causes severe neurological defects corresponding to the level at which the defect is found.

Children born with high lesions have a poor neurological prognosis and the majority of patients experience both bladder and bowel problems. For children with meningomyelocele a common complication is hydrocephalus. Owing to their immobility it is not unusual for these individuals to have many episodes of pressure sores (Figure 5.2).

Management

The management of pressure sores in children or teenagers with chronic illness or disability needs to address three important issues. These are:

Figure 5.2 *Teenager with spina bifida with a deep undermining pressure sore.*

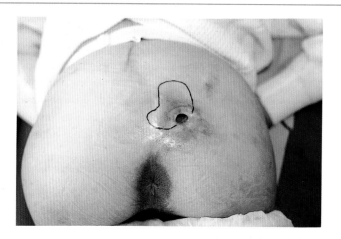

- Maintenance of self-care and independence
- Grants for pressure-relieving equipment
- Implications of pressure sores on the patient's general health and disability

It needs to be stressed that the effect of having a pressure sore will alter the whole lifestyle of the individual. Also the likelihood of further breakdown increases if adequate preventative measures are not put in place as a permanent part of management initially.

Multiple sore development over a period of time will cause further disability, require plastic surgery and predispose to life-threatening systemic infections.

The management of stage IV necrotic pressure sores is particularly problematic as the extent of the tissue damage under the necrotic eschar is often hidden. Damage may be superficial or may extend down to muscle and bone. This is a serious and potentially hazardous situation for a patient. Ninety per cent of elderly patients with such a pressure sore will die within 4 months (Bliss 1990). Debridement of this devitalized necrotic tissue can be achieved in several ways — surgically, chemically and by autolysis using dressings (see Chapter 8). Tracey may choose a conservative method of treatment which can be carried out at home by the district nurse. A hydrogel used with a semipermeable film in conjunction with sharp debridement of loose devitalized tissue is a common form of treatment.

For chairbound individuals the use of a written plan for the use of repositioning devices, negotiated between the individual and the professionals and tailored to the specific needs of the individual, is an effective way of reducing the likelihood of pressure sores (Van Etter *et al.* 1990). Included in this type of plan would be consideration of the postural alignment, distribution of weight, balance and stability, and pressure relief.

A seat cushion does much more than simply provide pressure relief. However, if the prescribed cushion interferes with daily activities of living and leisure then it is unlikely to be used. In addition to using an appropriate seat cushion, chairbound individuals can be taught to relieve pressure by shifting their weight regularly throughout the day. Relief of the high levels of pressure produced from sitting should be undertaken at least hourly. In patients with spinal cord injuries weight shifts have been shown to be effective in reducing the risk of pressure sores (Krouskop *et al.* 1983).

The care and management outlined below can be used as a framework for many individuals in similar situations.

Nursing model for Tracy

When assessing and planning Tracy's care the district nurse must be fully aware of Tracy's previous history. The nurse must also assess the family as a unit and not consider Tracy's needs apart from her family.

Although Tracy has a whole host of medical problems she also is an adolescent who has a right to be considered in all aspects of care (Muller *et al.* 1986).

Orem's model can assist the nurse in her assessment to instigate the development of family centred care. The nurse should be seen as the central 'facilitator' of care, not the main caregiver, and should be prepared to let go of tasks that may be seen traditionally as the nurse's.

The first stage of the assessment establishes whether there is a deficit in Tracy's self-care abilities. Remember, we are also assessing Tracy's mother as the main caregiver.

Orem's model uses six universal self-care needs to make the assessment (Table 5.3). Having identified Tracy's problems the nurse must decide why there is a self-care deficit. Is it due to a lack of knowledge, skills, motivation, or a limited range of behaviour? Tracy and her family were living a normal life before this period of hospitalization, and they may need to learn new skills or new behaviour in order to resume that normalcy. By recognizing the cause of the problem, the district nurse can plan with Tracy and her mother a new course of action which is suited to all concerned. The amount of intervention the nurse gives at this stage is crucial to the re-establishment of self-caring abilities.

Nursing intervention will be wholly compensatory, partly compensatory or educative/supportive (Table 5.4).

Table 5.3   *Assessment of Tracy (Case Study 5.2) using Orem's model*

Self-care need	Self-care ability	Self-care deficit
Sufficient intake of air	Tracy breathes without problems whichever position she is placed in	Nil
Fluid balance	Tracy is required to drink 2–3 litres daily to keep kidneys patent Feels weak following hospitalization	Needs extra fluids (A) Further urinary tract infection (P) Renal failure (P)
Nutrition	Extra energy needed owing to pressure sores and weight loss Tracy has never been a large eater	Weight loss (A) Catabolic state (A) Poor diet (A)
Elimination	Urostomy bag leaking due to weight loss and lying in bed Bowels evacuated daily by manual evacuation	Cannot manage urostomy without leakage (A) Diarrhoea due to antibiotics (P) Increase interface friction (P)
Activity and rest	Has had prolonged period in bed Will continue to spend more time in bed, not in wheelchair owing to pressure sores	Inadequate exercise (A) Muscle wasting (P) Non-healing pressure sores (A) Further skin breakdown (P)
Socializing	Normally a very sociable girl, Tracy has had a long period in hospital without her usual social contacts Mother has spent long periods in hospital with her	Depressed due to enforced hospitalization (A)
Normalcy	Normally goes to school Family outings Has friends to the house Considers her disability as normal to her	Missed schooling (A) Ill-health stopped family outings (A) Acute illness reinforces her disability (A)
Danger to self	Is able (with her mother's help) to manoeuvre herself in and out of bed and in and out of shower Feels weak and unable to perform normal hygiene or mobility roles	Further breakdown of skin (P) Chest infection (P) Injury to herself and mother (P)

(A), actual problem; (P), potential problem.

Table 5.4   *Nursing interventions for Tracy (Case Study 5.2)*

Self-care deficit	Goal	Interventions
a) Needs extra fluids (lack of skill and motivation) b) Further urinary tract infection	Tracy can drink as much as she can tolerate with an aim to reach 2 litres daily (PC)	a) Supply of Tracy's favourite drinks to be available at bedside in vacuum flasks or large juice containers. 'Bendy' straws or sealed containers will aid drinking when lying in bed
c) Renal failure (lack of knowledge)		b, c) Discuss level of knowledge of Tracy and her mother regarding the importance of keeping kidneys flushed with fluids. Use simple explanations without frightening them
a) Weight loss (limited range of behaviour)	To regain previous weight (PC)	a, b) Increase energy content of diet to enhance weight gain, but avoid protein overload of kidneys. Contact community dietician to plan specific diet with family. Discuss with Tracy and her mother effects of catabolism on wound healing
b) Catabolic state	To reduce the effects of catabolism and promote wound healing (PC, ES)	
c) Poor diet (lack of knowledge)	To promote a healthier diet for future eating (ES)	c) Plan a diet with the family which will take into account finances, availability of foodstuffs, and likes and dislikes.
a) Cannot manage urostomy bag (limited range of behaviour)	Eliminate leakage (WC)	a) Reassess urostomy bag size and stoma. Refer to stomatherapist for new appliance
b) Diarrhoea due to antibiotic (lack of knowledge)	Prevent diarrhoea and reduce interface friction (ES)	b) Explain importance of taking antibiotics at correct times. Advise Tracy to report any change in bowel motion
c) Increase of interface friction (lack of knowledge)		c) Reinforce importance of skin cleansing following urine spillage
a) Inadequate exercise (lack of motivation and limited behaviour)	To resume 'normal' physical activity level (PC, ES)	a, b) Resume daily routine of passive limits exercises of legs while in bed. Sit in chair for increasing periods each day, resuming arm lifts every half-hour. Discuss possibility of community physiotherapy weekly to keep motivation level high
b) Muscle wasting (limited behaviour)		
c) Non-healing pressure sores (lack of knowledge)	To heal pressure sores (WC) To prevent further sore development (ES)	c) Reassess Tracy using identified risk assessment tool and review whether pressure-relieving equipment (bed and chair) meets her needs
d) Further skin breakdown (lack of knowledge)		Document wound position, size and tissue characteristics. Trace and/or photograph. Debride wound, using dressing material that will i) keep wound occluded and prevent infection, ii) minimize dressing changes, iii) be possible for the mother to change if necessary, and iv) provide comfort for the patient d) Discuss with Tracy and her mother the reasons for initial sore development and indicators for prevention of future breakdown
a) Depressed owing to enforced hospitalization (lack of knowledge)	To introduce positive outlook on life (ES)	a) Encourage Tracy and her mother to reflect on the reasons why she went into hospital. Highlight the benefits of being home. Allow Tracy to work through her feelings, giving her time to talk

Table 5.4 *Continued*

Self-care deficit	Goal	Interventions
a) Missed schooling b) Family outings stopped c) Reinforcement of disability	To resume schooling and family routine (ES)	a) Arrange for social worker to investigate possibility of extra tuition b, c) Allow family to discuss difficulties of disablement and its effects on the family. Provide positive solutions. Look for indicators of family breakdown. Consider providing extra support for the family in the short term, e.g. a night sitter or day sitter
a) Further skin breakdown (lack of knowledge) b) Chest infection (lack of knowledge) c) Injury to Tracy or her mother (lack of knowledge)	To prevent further injury or disease to Tracy and her mother (ES)	a, c) Reinforce care of skin and lifting techniques a, c) Consider supplying equipment (hoist) as Tracy unable to lift as well as before b) Promote mobility, increasing the time spent in the wheelchair daily

ES, educative/supportive; PC, partly compensatory; WC, wholly compensatory.

Practice points

- In this case the district nurse's role has been mainly educative and partially compensatory. Even the wound care can be increasingly transferred to the mother.
- However, care must be taken that this role is willingly taken on. Often an acute episode like this triggers a breakdown in the family as the care unit.
- The nurse must assess the environment carefully and look for indications of strain and stress.

Road Traffic Accidents

Road traffic accidents are a common cause of traumatic wounds in teenagers, and the associated problems are illustrated in Case Study 5.3.

Case Study 5.3
Road traffic accident

Darren Adams had been employed as a motorbike courier for the last 6 months. Although he left school with 3 A-levels he was unable to find employment for 12 months. Despite the job being unsuited to his capabilities, he was pleased to have some form of income until the right job came along.

Darren has always liked drinking with his friends but has usually been sensible enough to walk or take a taxi home. Last Friday, however, it was raining heavily and he did not have any money left for a taxi so he decided to ride his bike home. The roads were slippery and at a junction Darren pulled out in front of a car. The car braked, but skidded into the bike, knocking Darren into the air some 2 metres before he landed on the bonnet of the car.

Darren was rushed to the local accident and emergency department. He was conscious, having sustained a fractured femur and severe lacerations to face and arm. Following admission Darren was informed that he was required to be interviewed by the police, at which point he became abusive and tried to throw himself off the trolley.

Epidemiology

In 1978 some 70 718 individuals in the UK were either killed or seriously injured in road traffic accidents (RoSPA 1989). Head injuries are more common in young males than females in a ratio of 3:1, mostly affecting the 16–35 age group. In the UK 5000 young people will be expected to die of their head injuries. In 1989 about 317 000 people were injured in road traffic accidents (Central Statistical Office 1990). It is sobering to realize that most of these injuries are preventable. The use of crash-helmets for motor-cyclists and safety belts in cars has resulted in less serious injuries. A common factor which contributes to head injuries is overconsumption of alcohol (Allan and Craig 1994).

Management

Many patients seen in accident and emergency departments are fit, young individuals. Irrespective of the wound size, accurate assessment, diagnosis and thorough wound toilet must be achieved in order that any deficit in wound healing is identified and the appropriate treatment given.

Before assessment of the traumatic wound is made patients must be stabilized. Standard assessments of airway, breathing and circulation are made to ensure that all life-threatening conditions are identified. Any external bleeding is controlled with direct pressure on the wound. A thorough history of how the accident happened is then recorded. This is limited by the conscious level of the patient if there are no accompanying witnesses. Other factors that are taken into account are:

- Exact mechanism of injury
- Amount of force
- Foreign bodies in wound
- Tendon or nerve damage
- Time and place of accident

It is important to establish whether the patient has any medical history of diabetes mellitus or epilepsy, is allergic or is taking any particular medication.

Wound assessment and cleansing

All traumatic wounds will be contaminated by the time the patient arrives in the accident and emergency department (Rodeheaver *et al.* 1974), therefore an aseptic technique is not necessary until removal of gross contaminants is achieved (Westaby and Thorn 1985). The following is recommended practice:

i)   Foreign material should be removed by washing (irrigation) (see Chapter 3), brushing or with forceps

ii) Before further investigation is attempted the wound must be anaesthetized with plain lignocaine

iii) Remove all deeply embedded foreign bodies and examine the damage in relation to underlying nerves and tendons (Evans 1991)

iv) Debridement of traumatized and devitalized tissue must be carried out, remembering that wound toilet should be directly proportional to the extent of contamination (Wound Healing Research Unit 1994).

Investigation

Radiographic investigations of traumatized limbs and suspected injury sites are required for an accurate diagnosis.

Antibiotics

Antibiotics are indicated for:

- Badly contaminated wounds
- Human or animal bites
- Diabetic or immunocompromised patients

Tetanus prophylaxis

Tetanus prophylaxis may be considered for wounds more than 6 hours old which display:

- Large amounts of devitalized tissue
- Deep puncture-type injury such as a stab wound
- Contact with soil or manure (e.g. in farm workers)
- Evidence of infection
- Human or animal bites (Wound Healing Research Unit 1994)

Nursing model for Darren

Darren has sustained major injuries and requires a great deal of immediate treatment. Unfortunately for him his arrival in the accident and emergency department has commenced with a confrontational event which is not conducive to developing a relationship with the nursing staff.

The nurse is required to calm Darren before commencing treatment and assessing his needs. The nurse may also need to consider the psychological consequences of labelling Darren as a drunken driver.

Darren has experienced a sudden change in circumstances from being a fit, healthy, intelligent young man. He is now immobile, facing criminal charges, and labelled as being stupid with no regard for other lives. In other words, he will need to adapt to ill-health. Roy's adaptation model (Roy 1980) may be used to assess and outline a plan of care (Table 5.5).

Table 5.5   *Assessment of Darren's problems (Case Study 5.3) using Roy's adaptation model*

Life area	Assessment Level 1 — Behaviour	Assessment Level 2 — Stimuli		
		Focal	*Contextual*	*Residual*
Self-concept	Abusive violent behaviour Fear of surroundings	Confrontation with A&E staff Still in shock	Staff not experienced in handling patient A&E department	Social stigma of drunk driver Never previously hospitalized
Role/function	Fears loss of job Fears police conviction	Major traumatic injury Knows he should not have driven	Extent of injury not assessed	No previous involvement with law
Interdependency	Dependent on staff, lack of self-control	Helpless owing to injuries and alcohol	Sudden change from being well to being seriously ill	Not 'normal' level of behaviour
Regulation	Multiple lacerations to face and arms Pain Contamination from road	Contaminated wounds Compound fracture of femur Infection in wound	Wounds embedded with grit and dirt from road Further damage to underlying tissue Length of time before arrival in A&E	
Oxygenation	Hyperventilation	Fear and shock	Pain in leg	
Nutrition	Feeling nauseated	Pin in leg Shock	Effects of alcohol	

Practice points

- Before Darren can have an assessment of his traumatic injuries the staff need to calm him as he is in grave danger of adding to his injuries.

- Look at the assessment of his psychosocial status and identify the major problems:
  - violent behaviour due to *shock fear* and effects of *alcohol*
  - placed in hospital surroundings which are *new* to him
  - does not have any *family or friends* to provide *support*

How can these problems be resolved?

Because of the way in which the traumatic injuries are incurred, patients are suddenly plunged into what may seem a hostile environment in the accident and emergency unit. This is compounded in Darren's case as the police are also there waiting to see him.

Darren's wounds were debrided, irrigated and sutured. Antibiotic cover and frequent wound observation were instituted for the prevention and early detection of wound infection. In the long term the extent of Darren's scarring could have a lasting effect on his psychological state. Facial wounds often require the skills of a plastic surgeon using careful suturing techniques (see Chapter 4).

Most accident and emergency departments operate a triage system, enabling staff to prioritize patient care. Those requiring immediate emergency treatment are attended to first, while less urgent cases are dealt with later. In this case it might have been advisable to assess Darren's injuries and gain his confidence before the police were mentioned.

The priority of management is to ensure there are no life-threatening problems by using the 'ABC' protocol (airway, breathing and circulation), checking that there are no major bleeding points at the site of fracture, and assessing previous blood loss. Check vital signs for signs of shock. Calm the patient with:

- Reassurance — talk slowly, in a quiet area away from the hustle and bustle of the department. Enlist his trust, the nurse is there to help him.
- Pain relief — give appropriate analgesia, if vital signs are satisfactory. Local analgesia may also be required before wound toilet is commenced at site of fracture.
- Explanation — explain the necessity to assess his injuries as quickly as possible and that this will require his coperation. Ask him if he would like his family contacted.

Accident and emergency department staff are trained to provide reassurance and gain the patient's trust quickly, while simultaneously performing resuscitation techniques.

Look at the physiological areas of assessment. The important points here are:

- Wound cleansing and wound toilet
- Thorough examination of lacerations and extent of injuries
- Antibiotic and tetanus cover
- Accurate documentation of both events of accident and nature of injury

Devise the care plan, taking these points into account. Look at the assessment in Table 5.5 if you need help.

Summary

Injury to teenagers can be traumatic both physiologically and psychologically. The nurse has an important role to play in providing skilled management of the wound and gaining the patient's trust. The bond that can develop between nurse and teenager can be rewarding and enhance the level of care given.

The important issues to remember when dealing with the cases outlined can be summarized as follows:

■ gain the trust of the teenager before commencement of any treatment

■ ensure there is always adequate pain relief given

■ consider the effects that immobility or scarring may have on them for the rest of their lives

■ be aware that teenagers can easily be emotionally crushed; always communicate in a clear and understanding way

■ documentation, as always, is of utmost importance. Claims may be made many years on from the actual date of the accident or injury

■ be aware that inadequate management may result in inadequate wound healing

Further Reading

Wardrope J & Smith J (1993) *The Management of Wounds and Burns*. Oxford University Press.

Salter M (1988) *Altered Body Image*. London: Scutari.

Gowar JP & Lawrence JC (1995) The incidence, cause and treatment of minor burns. *Journal of Wound Care* 4(2): 71–74.

Howe J (1980) *Nursing Care of Adolescents*. New York: McGraw-Hill.

Wright B (1993) *Caring in Crisis: A handbook of Intervention Skills*, 2nd edn. Edinburgh: Churchill Livingstone.

Wright LM & Leahy M (1987) *Families and clinical illness*. Springhouse, Penn: Springhouse.

Walsh M (1990) *Accident and Emergency Nursing. A New Approach*, 2nd edn. Oxford: Butterworth-Heinemann.

References

Allan D & Craig E (1994) The nervous system. In: Alexander MR, Fawcett JN & Runciman PJ (eds) *Nursing Practice*. Edinburgh: Churchill Livingstone.

Bliss M (1990) Geriatric medicine. In: Bader DL (ed.) *Pressure Sores. Clinical Practice and Scientific Approach*, Chapter 7. London: Macmillan.

British Paediatric Association (1989) *The Needs and Care of Adolescents*. Report of BPA Working Party. London: BPA.

Central Statistical Office (1990) *Annual Abstract of Statistics*. London: HMSO.

Central Statistical Office (1991) *Social Trends*. No 21. London: HMSO.

Evans R (1991) Pitfalls in traumatic wound care. *Wound Management* 1(1): 8–10.

Farrelly R (1994) The special care needs of adolescents in hospital. *Nursing Times* 90(38): 31–33.

Gillies M (1992) Teenage traumas. *Nursing Times* 88(27): 26–29.

Krouskop TA, Noble PL, Garber SL & Spencer WA (1983) The effectiveness of preventative management in reducing the occurrence of pressure sores. *Journal of Rehabilitation* 20(1): 74–83.

Lawrence JC (1990) *Burn and Scald Injuries*. Topic Briefing HS40. Birmingham: RoSPA.

Muller D, Harris PJ & Wattley LA (1986) *Nursing Children: Psychology Research and Practice*. London: Harper & Row.

Neale AB & Haine CV (1983) *Birminghan Statistics 1981–82*. City of Birmingham Centre Statistics Office.

Petch N & Cason CG (1993) Examining first aid received by burn and scald patients. *Journal of Wound Care* 2(2): 102–105.

Rodeheaver GP, Pettry D & Turnbull V (1974) Identification of the wound infection — potentiating factors in soil. *American Journal of Surgery* 128: 8–14.

Roper N, Logan WW & Tierney AJ (1980) *The Elements of Nursing*. Edinburgh: Churchill Livingstone.

RoSPA (1989) *Child Safety in the Home*. Home Safety Topic Guide. Birmingham: RoSPA.

Roy C (1980) The Roy adaptation model. In: Riehl JP & Roy C (eds) *Conceptual Models for Nursing Practice*. 2nd edn. New York: Appleton-Century-Crofts.

Settle JAD (1986) *Burns — the First Five Days*. Smith & Nephew Pharmaceuticals Ltd.

Van Etter NK, Sexton P & Smith R (1990) Development and implementation of a skin care program. *Ostomy Wound Management* March–April 27: 40–54.

Weller B (1985) *Paediatric Nursing Practice and Techniques*. London: Harper & Row.

Westaby S & Thorn A (1985) Treatment of wounds in A&E Dept. In: Westaby S (ed.) *Wound Care*. London: Heinemann.

Wijetunge D (1992) An accident and emergency approach. *Journal of Wound Management* Nursing Supplement. *Nursing Times* 88(46): 70–76.

Wound Healing Research Unit (1994) *Wound Management — Good Practice Guidance*. NHS Cymru, Wales.

6

Wound Care in the Young Adult

Key issues

This chapter examines the type of wound management required by the young adult.

Clinical Case Studies

Aetiology and management of:

- A 22-year-old man requiring emergency excision of pilonidal sinus
- A woman requiring an emergency caesarean section who encounters wound problems post-operatively
- Post-operative care of a woman following elective surgery for hidradenitis suppurativa
- A 34-year-old mother with osteosarcoma of the leg
- A leg wound inflicted by the patient

Nursing Models

Examples of their application to practice are taken from:

- Orem's model
- Roy's adaptation model
- Riehl's interaction model

Practice points

As you read through this chapter concentrate on the following:

- The effects emergency surgery may have on post-operative wound management.
- Factors that should be considered in pre-operative management that enhance post-operative care.
- The effect a wound can have on the normal living pattern of patients.
- The range of dressings available that patients can manage themselves.
- The importance of including the patient in planning care.

Introduction

Young adulthood is a stage in the life-cycle where the individual feels immune to disease and ill-health. The young value their youthfulness and vigour and generally thrive on fitness. For the young the image of a sick individual may be one of a helpless, older person being the passive recipient of both medical and nursing care. This age group would challenge this image and feel confident, empowered and expect to become involved in making decisions about their care and management. The Patients' Charter (Department of Health 1991) actively seeks to promote the nurse and patient working together in partnership, giving the patients an opportunity to make informed choices about their care. Nurses should bear this in mind when dealing with young adults and also take into account their opinions.

Preparing for Planned Surgery

Surgical procedures may be offered to many young people with a variety of health problems. For many problems that are not life-threatening the decision to accept or refuse surgery rests solely with the individual. Examples of these problems include lipomas and ingrowing toenails; the patient will decide how troublesome it is. Other health problems such as inguinal hernia, ovarian cyst and pilonidal sinus may lead to further complications and are best treated with surgical intervention. Individuals vary greatly in their response to the prospect of surgery: some regard it in a matter-of-fact way, others with great fear and trepidation. Experiences in childhood or the experiences of family members or friends can be an influencing factor.

Great advances have been made in surgical procedures. The use of the laparoscope for 'keyhole' surgery has enabled knee surgery and abdominal surgery to be carried out through very small incisions. Where appropriate, such operations can take place in day surgery units where the patient need not stay overnight. From a cost-saving point of view, there is an increasing trend for young, fit individuals to be offered day surgery. From the patient's point of view the advantages include a short stay in hospital, reduced pain and immobility, and an earlier return to normal activities.

Patients requiring more extensive surgery will need to be admitted to a surgical ward. Pre-operatively the nurse has an important role to play in helping to prepare the patient for surgery. As well as the physical assessment the nurse can provide information and emotional support on admission. It is well documented that with information and support given to reduce stress and anxiety, the patient has a much better post-operative outcome (Rodgers 1994).

With planning, education need not be disrupted, and it is usual for young patients to be offered a date for surgery to coincide with college holidays. Interruption of daily activities may be perceived as problematic for the young individual. Concern may be focused around the length of time that a favourite sport may not be played, or when they may be able to go out socially. Linked to this may be concerns for the young person of an altered body image. The young value their youth, health, beauty and vigour

(Smitherman 1981) and any disfigurement, however minor, may have a negative effect.

Coping with Emergency Surgery

The onset of an acute illness or trauma can result in the need for emergency surgery. An example is given in Case Study 6.1. Preparation of the young person as described above may not be possible, and often only brief, essential information can be given in the immediate pre-operative period. In the post-operative period patients are likely to have many questions, which could need answering several times as the patient recovers from both the anaesthesia and surgery.

Case Study 6.1

Emergency excision of pilonidal sinus

Colin Sharples is a 22-year-old law student just entering his final year of studies. A fit, healthy young man who has always been involved in many sporting activities, he has never had any experience of illness or hospitalization.

During the past 6 months he has had a feeling of discomfort in his natal cleft which appears to come and go and is often associated with feeling generally unwell. Last week the discomfort became an acute, stabbing pain which prevented him from sitting down. He went to the college doctor who diagnosed his condition as pilonidal disease and gave him a course of antibiotics. Colin unfortunately took his antibiotics for 2 days only as he felt better and did not really like taking tablets. Within a week he was admitted to hospital for an emergency wide excision of a pilonidal abscess.

Following surgery the wound was left to heal by secondary intention, and measured 10 cm in length by 3 cm breadth and 4 cm depth. Colin was extremely anxious post-operatively and, although in pain, was reluctant to stay in hospital as he wanted to resume his studies.

Aetiology

Pilonidal sinus disease commonly affects young adults, arising at some time after puberty. More than 7000 patients were admitted for an average of 5 days to English hospitals for treatment (Office of Population Censuses and Surveys data). This is indeed a disease of the young adult with most patients becoming clear of this disease by about the age of 40 years (Haywood and Clothier 1984). Pilonidal sinus disease causes a great deal of suffering, inconvenience, loss of time from work and loss of income, as patients can have problems for at least 3 years (Clothier and Haywood 1985). The recurrence rate following surgery can be as high as 50% (Jones 1992).

There are several theories as to why pilonidal sinus disease occurs, the most likely being acquired disease (Figure 6.1). With the onset of puberty, sex hormones begin to act on pilosebaceous glands in the natal cleft. With this a hair follicle becomes distended with **keratin** and subsequently infected, so resulting in a folliculitis and an abscess which extends down into

Keratin
an insoluble protein forming the principal component of epidermis, hair, nails and tooth enamel

Figure 6.1 *(a) Pilonidal sinus; (b) pilonidal abscess; (c) a combination of pilonidal sinus with pilonidal abscess.*

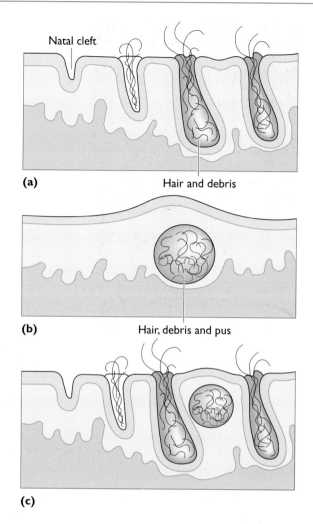

Natal cleft

(a)   Hair and debris

(b)   Hair, debris and pus

(c)

subcutaneous fat. In 93% the direction of the abscess and secondary tracts follows the orientation of the inflamed hair follicles. The abscess is likely to drain out onto the skin through the tract (Berry 1992). Hairs are drilled or sucked into the abscess cavity through friction with movement of the buttocks. This process encourages loose debris and other body hair to enter and accumulate in the sinus (Figure 6.2). Most commonly *Staphylococcus aureus* and *Bacteroides* are the pathogens causing the infection. Patients may be asymptomatic for some time before presenting with local discomfort and/or discharge. However, about 50% of patients present with an acute pilonidal abscess.

Management

Several treatments may be offered to patients:-

- Curettage for small, non-infected sinuses; it may be possible to remove the hairs with a pair of forceps and to clean out the track.

Figure 6.2 *Pilonidal sinus disease prior to surgery. Marked on the patient's skin is the area to be excised, together with the sites of individual sinuses.*

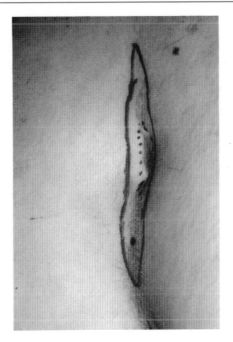

- Excision and primary closure — here the sinuses are excised and the wound edges brought together and sutured.
- Wide excision and laying open of the sinuses together with the skin; all tissues are excised down to the sacrum. The patient requires frequent dressing changes and a great deal of support. The advantages of performing more radical surgery is the low recurrence rate associated with it, of 1% at 1 year (Wood *et al.* 1972).

As Colin's disease was widespread the wide excision technique was used leaving a large cavity wound (Figures 6.3 to 6.6).

Local Wound Management

This large cavity will take about 6–8 weeks to heal by secondary intention. With a little care Colin could return to fairly normal activities quickly and could take responsibility for his own wound hygiene. Some of the dressing materials that could be used include:

- Day 0–2 — alginate materials, especially those containing sodium, are useful haemostatic agents. The dressing can be packed into the wound immediately following surgery, in the operating theatre, to achieve haemostasis. After 48 hours this alginate packing can be washed out of the cavity using warm saline.
- Day 2 through the proliferative phase — alginate materials can be used, but this treatment needs a nurse to change the dressings. Other useful

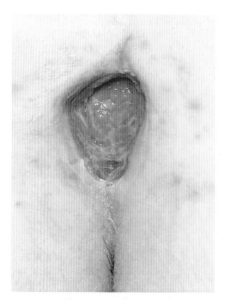

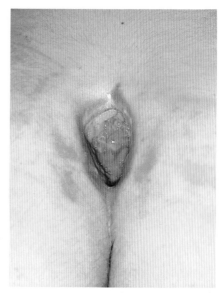

Figure 6.3   *Wide excision of pilonidal sinus at week 2.*

Figure 6.4   *At week 4.*

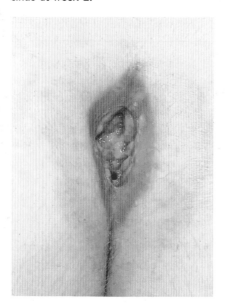

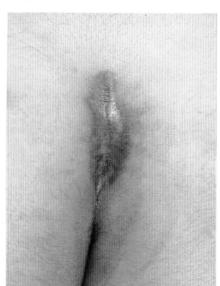

Figure 6.5   *At week 6.*

Figure 6.6   *At week 8 – healed.*

materials include cavity foam dressings and occasionally a hydrogel. Foam dressings, especially those formed in situ, can be managed by patients on a daily basis and so facilitate early return to normal activity. The main functions of a cavity dressing for a pilonidal sinus excision is to keep the wound edges apart as healing takes place, so preventing superficial bridges and the possibility of a dead space in the depths of the wound.

Nursing model for Colin

Colin is a normal, fit, healthy young adult who does not really want to be in hospital or have his normal routine altered. What do you see as his main concerns?

- Disruption of his studies
- Disruption of his sporting activities
- Disruption of sexual activity
- Embarrassment at exposing buttocks to nurses
- Lack of privacy in hospital
- Likelihood of recurrence of disease
- Time of discharge from hospital

Colin's major worries are not directly concerned with wound management. In a fit, healthy young man this open granulating wound should heal easily and without complication.

Practice points

You should have identified Colin's self-care deficit from the list of main concerns. The management that Colin needs, therefore, should follow these lines:

- Following an initial 3–4 days in hospital Colin can be discharged with arrangements made with the community nurse or university campus nurse to arrange care.
- Initially the wound could be packed with alginates to achieve haemostasis; then, in the next few days, a cavity foam dressing could be introduced. Colin could change these dressings himself, following daily showering. He needs to understand that strenuous exercise must be avoided for up to 12 weeks.
- Colin requires a flexible approach to his care, the need to feel in control and the assurance that he has professional advice when needed.
- Orem's model would fulfil these needs, with an early discharge into the community under the care of the university campus nurse and specialist outpatient visits at frequent intervals.

Caesarean Section

Case Study 6.2 discusses the problems arising from wound breakdown after an apparently straightforward caesarean section.

Case Study 6.2
Caesarean section

Mrs Kate Hemmings, a 34-year-old, gave birth to her third child by emergency caesarean section. Kate had a caesarean delivery with her first child, but delivered her second child normally and had wanted to try and deliver this baby normally also. Following 7 days in hospital Kate and baby Julia were discharged home into the care of the community staff.

Her sutures were removed at 10 days with the wound apparently having healed without any complications. She felt well in herself, albeit a little tired, but felt this was to be expected with a small baby and two other toddlers to cope with.

By the 12th day she noticed a small red spot in the middle of the scar line which, following a bath, began to ooze fluid. Alarmed at this, she called the district nurse who placed a dressing pad on the offending area.

Over the next week the oozing continued and an opening became visible which measured 2 cm in width when probed. The surrounding wound area was hard and red and she was feeling generally unwell. The district nurse probed the wound and found it undermined 1 cm either side of the scar line (Figure 6.7). The nurse called the general practitioner who admitted Kate to the gynaecology ward at the local hospital. The wound was opened up 1.5 cm either side of the gaping edge to make a small cavity to facilitate drainage of exudate (Figures 6.8 to 6.10). The wound was packed with an alginate dressing, and on Kate's insistence she was discharged home 48 hours later.

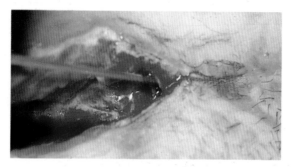

Figure 6.7   *Kate Hemmings' wound, showing a probe inserted into the undermining area.*

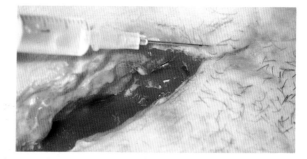

Figure 6.8   *Local anaesthetic being injected into the area to be incised.*

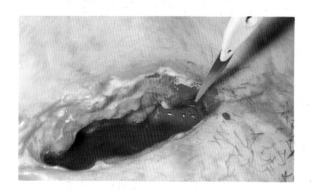

Figure 6.9   *Incising the undermined area.*

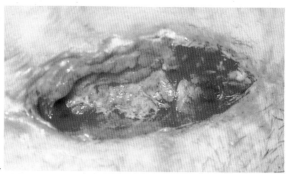

Figure 6.10   *The resultant cavity wound is now a suitable shape for healing by secondary intention.*

Aetiology

Caesarean section is the operation by which a potentially viable fetus is delivered through an incision in the abdominal wall and uterus. One of the earliest records of a caesarean section being performed on a viable fetus dates from around 140 BC. The incidence of caesarean section has gradually risen in the UK to around 10% of deliveries, and is likely to increase with the problems of litigation linked to complicated, prolonged vaginal deliveries.

The most common surgical technique employed is the lower segment caesarean section (Figure 6.11). Here an incision is made over the lower uterine segment, which is less vascular than the upper segment so reducing the risk of bleeding. Post-operative infection is also reduced because the lower segment is outside the peritoneal cavity.

Management

Normally wound management would entail removal of sutures between 10–14 days. Here, however, as with breakdown of surgical wounds, it is advisable to incise the wound to allow free drainage of exudate (see Chapter 3).

This type of wound can be managed using an alginate packing dressing, gently inserted into the undermining wound. The function of the dressing in this situation is to maintain a channel through which infected exudate can drain and to allow the wound to heal from its depths. It is probably advisable to irrigate the cavity daily with water or saline, prior to repacking. This will rinse out any fragments of alginate left in the wound and also flush away bacteria. Alternatively, a hydrogel could be introduced into the wound to act as packing. Again, daily irrigation would be beneficial.

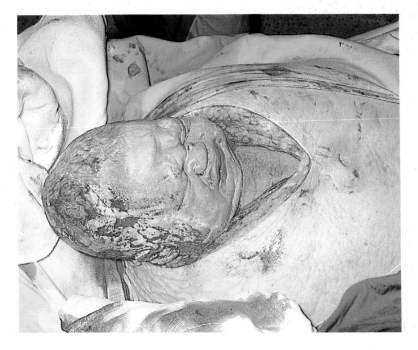

Figure 6.11 *The lower uterine segment has been excised transversely and the large fetal head, directly occipitoposterior, has been delivered by manual extraction.*

Nursing model for Kate

It is obvious that Kate has a post-operative wound infection which requires immediate treatment. However, having had to leave her baby, two young children and husband at home, she insisted on returning home within 48 hours.

It is important to provide her with a flexible form of management that allows her to cope at home. She needs to feel in control of her own care, but obviously requires support both emotionally and physically from family and health professions.

Before choosing a model of care, ask yourself the following questions:

- Will Kate be able, or want, to do the dressing herself?
- How will the presence of the wound infection affect the young baby?
- What were the possible reasons for her developing this infection?
- Why is it better that Kate stays at home during her recovery?

Orem's model (Orem 1980) would address Kate's problems, as she will probably be motivated to achieve self-care (Table 6.1).

Table 6.1   *Assessment of Mrs Hemmings' problems (Case Study 6.2) using Orem's model*

Self-care need	Self-care ability	Self-care deficit
Nutrition	Little time to eat with three children Little appetite owing to infection Losing nutrients through breast-feeding	Inadequate diet (A) Anaemia (P) Unable to breast-feed (P)
Activity and rest	Not sleeping because of new baby Worried infection will be passed to baby	Delay in wound healing due to lack of sleep (A) Unable to play with children and baby
Socializing	Unable to go out with baby owing to wound infection	Depression (P) No normal mother–baby activities (A)
Normalcy	Needs to wait in for nurse to do dressings	Feels restricted Cannot get into routine with other children and baby

(A), actual problem; (P), potential problem.

Practice point

You must plan the management in such a way that Kate can resume her way of life as quickly as possible.

Hidradenitis Suppurativa

The unpleasant symptoms of hidradenitis suppurativa drive patients to seek surgical intervention, as in the example in Case Study 6.3.

Case Study 6.3
Elective excision of hidradenitis suppurativa

Mrs Hannah Mitchell is a married woman of 36 years of age with three children aged 10, 7 and 3. Most of her adult life she has suffered with repeated abscesses and boils in both axillae.

Her condition was diagnosed 8 years ago as hidradenitis suppurativa but, owing to pregnancy, breast-feeding, and general child-rearing commitments, she has been unable until now to present herself for surgical excision of the offending sweat glands.

Although she had endured years of pain and discomfort and various courses of antibiotics, she remained anxious at the thought of the pain after the operation and the type of scarring that she might be left with. Fortunately she was able to meet someone who had previously been operated on, see the finished result and discuss any anxieties.

During her proposed stay Hannah had organized the child-care arrangements between her mother and husband who had taken 2 weeks off work.

The operation went well and following removal of the post-operative dressing Hannah had bilateral axillae wounds measuring 15 cm long by 6 cm wide and 3 cm deep. Pregranulation tissue was healthy and the wound was draining large amounts of exudate. Removal of the alginate packs was uncomfortable even though 75 mg of pethidine had been administered intramuscularly 30 minutes beforehand.

Aetiology

Abscess
a collection of pus which has localized. It is formed by the liquefactive disintegration of tissue and a large accumulation of polymorphonuclear leucocytes

Hidradenitis suppurativa is a chronic inflammatory condition of the skin and subcutaneous tissues occurring in areas where apocrine sweat glands are found. Apocrine sweat glands are found mainly in the axillae, groin and perineal areas, but are also found in the labia, scrotum, lower back, and in and around the breasts. This disease is characterized by deep, painful **abscesses** which erupt through the skin draining pus. Abscess formation continues over a period of years and is associated with cellulitis, sinus formation and subcutaneous tunnelling. Adolescence often marks the onset of hidradenitis suppurativa and patients are incapacitated by this distressing disease over a number of years before presenting for surgical treatment. In one study the time from onset of this disease to receiving surgery ranged from 1 year to 42 years, with a mean of 9 years (Harrison *et al.* 1988). The cause of this disease is largely unknown, but women are twice as likely to be affected. Hormonal activity and endocrine disorders have been reported to affect symptoms (Harrison *et al.* 1988).

These young patients are often managed conservatively with long-term, low-dose antibiotic treatment or by multiple local excision of individual abscesses. As years pass the patient's quality of life is generally affected by these recurrent boils and abscesses. The young person is often embarrassed by abscesses draining and the associated malodour. Pain can be severe in the affected area, leading to disruption of school, college or work. The forming

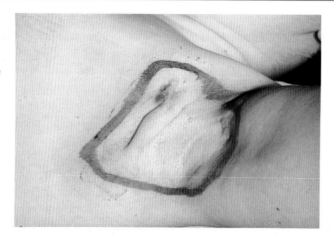

Figure
6.12 *Hidradenitis suppurativa of the axilla preoperatively showing the affected axilla and the extent of tissue to be excised.*

of interpersonal and sexual relationships can be severely disrupted, with the young person missing out on the normal social activities which their peers take for granted. A combination of these factors prompts the individual to seek surgical intervention. However, surgical excision of hidradenitis suppurativa is not undertaken lightly. To be effective, all the skin bearing diseased apocrine sweat glands needs to be excised, with the extent of the excision being determined by the extent of the disease (Figure 6.12). The decision to undergo extensive surgery should be made by the patient after being counselled about the extent of the surgery, the cosmetic results, the immediate post-operative expectations and the long-term prospects. Owing to the severe morbidity experienced by patients with this disease, many young patients elect to have extensive surgery.

Management

Following surgical excision of the affected skin and subcutaneous tissues, the wounds are packed for 48–72 hours to achieve haemostasis; haemostatic alginate dressings are useful for this purpose. As the wound is extensive, copious amounts of wound exudate are produced. A comfortable, soft, absorbent, practical dressing that can be used throughout the healing phase is a silicone-based foam which is poured into the wound to form a stent, which is a reusable dressing. When used by skilled practitioners the dressings do not require surgical tape to hold them in place. A combination of a well-formed dressing, the patient's clothing and absorbent dressing pads holds the dressing in contact with the wound. Not using tape is an important consideration, as the wound is likely to take up to 3 months to heal. Patients usually spend less than 2 weeks in hospital and are encouraged to return gradually to normal activity. Where silicone dressings are used, patients can be taught to perform their own dressing changes and wound cleansing. With this type of reusable dressing this is best carried out twice a day to help reduce the bacterial load of the dressings to an acceptable level. Teaching patients to care for their own wounds in this way requires help and support

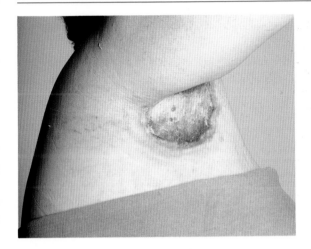

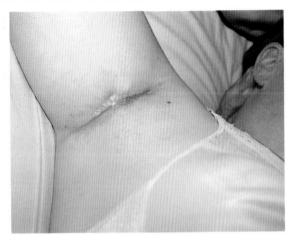

Figure 6.13 *Hannah Mitchell at week 2 showing healthy granulation tissue and some re-epithelialization.*

Figure 6.14 *At week 9, the wound is healed, showing a good cosmetic affect with linear scarring.*

both from the community nurses and the hospital where the surgery took place. Although these young patients are pleased to be able to return home, there are considerable costs to be incurred in obtaining dressings over a long period of time on prescription from the general practitioner. It may be advisable for patients not exempt from paying prescription charges to apply for a 3-month or 6-month season ticket to cover these costs. One payment purchases a certificate which covers all prescription charges for that period.

In the immediate post-operative period movement is likely to be difficult and painful, but as time passes this will dramatically improve. Physiotherapy and gentle movements will prevent wound contractures, the resultant scar being approximately 10% of the original wound. Generally patients are happy with the scar, with 91% sufficiently satisfied that they would wish to undergo the procedure again (Harrison 1988) (Figures 6.13 and 6.14).

Nursing model for Hannah

Look back at Hannah's case. What are the important features that stand out about this patient?

- She has *endured pain* and distress for many years
- She has *dependent children*
- She has *waited* a long time for this operation
- She *needs/wants* to go *home*
- She has *limited* range of *movement*

Practice point

From these points, what can you assume about the type of care the patient needs?

Hannah needs to go home, but will require much support from the community nurses. She is a strong, determined woman, therefore problems could develop if she chooses not to follow the community nurse's advice on wound care.

Peplau (1952) recognized the care the patient needs may be different from what he or she wants. Peplau's assessment (orientation) could be used by the district nurse, as follows:

- The nurse learns the nature of the difficulty the patient is experiencing
- The nurse and patient develop a mutual trust
- The nurse can then identify the patient's problems

Practice point

Using the SOAP assessment framework (Chapter 2), plan Hannah's care.

Malignant Tumours

The problems of terminal disease are discussed in relation to an unsuccessfully treated osteosarcoma (Case Study 6.4).

Case Study 6.4
Osteosarcoma of the tibia

Fungate
to produce fungus-like growths; to grow rapidly

Fiona Starr, a 34-year-old mother of two small children, has osteosarcoma of the tibia and is in the terminal stages of the disease.

Following diagnosis 18 months ago Fiona decided on a course of chemotherapy and radiotherapy rather than a below-knee amputation. Initially the treatment appeared successful and the tumour shrank in size. Unfortunately, 6 months ago the tumour reappeared with a vengeance and despite a further course of chemotherapy, began to **fungate** and ulcerate.

The whole of the lower leg is now affected with a fungating mass, is swollen due to lymphoedema and is painful to touch (Figure 6.15). The malignancy has infiltrated to the lymphatic system and there is involvement of the organs of the pelvic region.

Fiona has chosen to be nursed in a hospice setting where her family have free access. She is fully aware of her prognosis but has difficulty coming to terms with her initial decision of refusing surgery, as this would probably have halted the disease process.

Figure 6.15 *Fungating osteosarcoma of the tibia.*

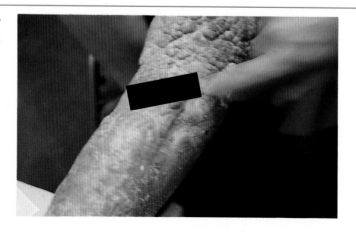

Aetiology

Malignant tumours are made up of cells which are able to invade adjacent tissues but are also able to leave the original site and disseminate to other areas and form metastases. There are three major groups of cancers:

- Carcinomas — arise in endodermal or ectodermal tissue
- Sarcomas — mesodermal in origin
- Leukaemias/lymphomas — derived from white blood cells and the monocyte-macrophage system

Osteosarcoma most commonly occurs in the lower end of the femur, the upper end of the tibia or the upper end of the humerus. These tumours occur in young people and present as swelling of the affected area with or without vague aching. A plain X-ray film shows an increase in radiolucency associated with bone expansion, triangular areas of new bone formation at the periosteal margin and a 'sunray' appearance due to new bone being formed (Macleod *et al.* 1987). Metastases are rapidly blood-borne to the lung, and the survival rate at 5 years is likely to be less than 10%. As the disease progresses the cancer may spread into the lymphatic system and also ulcerate through the skin to form a fungating mass. Malodour, increased exudate production, bleeding or fear of bleeding and asymmetry are common problems caused by the fungating mass.

Management

The young person may feel socially isolated and experience altered body image and sexual difficulties as a result. The skilful use of dressing materials can cope with the physical problems of odour, bleeding and excess exudate. Bleeding can be controlled with haemostatic alginate dressings and odour can be controlled with topical use of metronidazole gel which quickly and effectively acts against anaerobic organisms. It can be applied daily at dressing changes until the odour is no longer noticeable. Charcoal dressings absorb odour but need to be held in close contact with the wound or primary dressing to be effective. At a palliative level these physical symptoms can be managed. The psychological issues are far more difficult to deal with. Impending death is not an easy issue for the young, and the interaction between the patient, the family and the professional team is of vital importance.

Nursing model for Fiona

The demands placed on Fiona and on those who care for her during her illness require special assessment from the nurse in order to provide the right type of care. Roy's adaptation model (Roy 1980) is designed to help the nurse identify the patient's problems and promote the patient's ability to adapt and cope with them.

Look at one of Fiona's adaptation systems as identified by Roy — the *self-concept system*. This is the view the individual holds of herself both physically and psychologically. What problems of adaptation do you think she has?

Table 6.2 lists some of the stressors causing problems. Look next at the level 2 assessment in Table 6.3 — which are caused by focal, contextual or residual stimuli.

Table 6.2   *Assessment of Fiona Starr's self-concept system (Case Study 6.4)*

Life area	Assessment Level I — Behaviour
Self-concept a) Physical	i) Cannot look at the swollen, fungating, malodorous leg ii) Cannot get away from wound — constantly living (dying) with it

b) Psychological	i) Feelings of guilt, e.g.
	   depriving family of mother and wife
	   should have chosen other treatment option
	ii) Loss of body image and feelings of mutilation

Table 6.3   *Level 2 assessment of Fiona Starr*

Assessment Level I — Behaviour	Assessment Level 2 — Stimuli		
	Focal	Contextual	Residual
a(i)*	Odour Lymphoedema Fungation	Nursed away from other patients Dressings not suited to wound	May have previous experience of seeing dying patients with wounds
a(ii)	Frequent dressing changes	Nurses' attitude when performing dressing changes	Previous information given about progress of wound
b(i)	Children and husband upset at Fiona's condition	Hospice setting and attitude of staff to Fiona	Information given at previous treatment consultations

* See Table 6.2.

Practice points

- The management of the wound must focus around the stimuli causing her particular behaviour.
- Fiona needs counselling to adapt her behaviour to a more balanced view to help her and her family cope.

- She needs to talk through her treatment decisions and come to terms with why she made the decision she did.

- What particular wound management could she have that would help her to adapt?

Factitious Wounds

Factitious or self-inflicted wounds can pose enormous problems to healthcare staff, as shown in Case Study 6.5.

Case Study 6.5
Self-inflicted injury

Justina Finlay has presented to her general practitioner with an area of necrotic tissue above the inside of her left ankle.

On examination the wound is 4 cm in diameter with a surrounding area of inflamed tissue. The general practitioner does not know Justina very well, but takes only a brief history and sends her to the practice nurse for a dressing.

Justina does not go into the practice nurse's treatment room that day but presents herself 3 days later in a somewhat anxious state. Sister Andrews, an experienced nurse who has worked both in general nursing and psychiatry, sits Justina down and before looking at her wound spends some time asking her about her medical and social history.

Justina is unemployed and lives in a small caravan with some friends on the outskirts of the town. She states that she cut her ankle while chopping wood and had tried to dress it herself, but that it has gone septic-looking and now black.

Examination of the wound revealed widespread cellulitis and phlebitis surrounding an obviously infected, necrotic wound (Figure 6.16). Sister Andrews attempted mechanical debridement of the wound but this was too painful, and Justina became agitated and threatened to leave the surgery. The nurse measured Justina's temperature (which was 39.5°C) and blood pressure: while doing so she noticed needle marks covering the arm.

Figure 6.16 *Justina Finlay's ankle showing self-inflicted wound following intravenous drug abuse.*

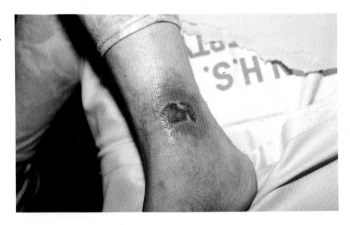

Aetiology

It is a common assumption by clinicians that the shared goal or outcome for both the patient with a wound and the professionals caring for that patient is to achieve healing of the wound (Baragwanath *et al.* 1994a). However, for a small percentage of patients this is not the case, and individuals are responsible for either creating a wound or preventing an existing wound from healing. Identifying these patients is difficult and their wound treatment very often ineffective (Drinker *et al.* 1972). One study established the incidence of factitious wounds as being 0.5% of non-healing wounds attending a specialist wound clinic (Baragwanath *et al.* 1994b). This study reported that although the mean age at which patients received treatment for their factitious wounds was 44 years, the mean age of onset of the wounds was much lower at 34 years, with equal numbers of men and women presenting. Young patients had a particular set of social circumstances thought to be associated with their psychotic illness. All young people were single and still living at home with their parents. For this young group of patients the average age of onset of the non-healing wound was 20 years, and these individuals demonstrated limited social maturity and found difficulties in forming personal relationships outside their family group. Some young people with factitious injury fail to take responsibility for their own life and use their wound as an excuse to remain at home and be dependent on their family (Lyell 1972). As this illness progresses the young individual becomes increasingly socially isolated and dependent on both family and healthcare professionals. Should the true nature of the non-healing wound be suspected and the patient confronted, denial is likely to be rapidly followed by the patient seeking referral to another healthcare professional (Fras and Coughlin 1972).

Although tempting, direct confrontation is not an effective approach for young individuals with factitious wounds. An alternative approach has been put forward (Baragwanath *et al.* 1994a, Eisedrath 1989). Here the nurse or doctor informs the patient that they know what might have caused the wound not to heal, but also, at the same time, offers an alternative explanation. A new wound treatment is then prescribed and the patient is told that if this new treatment is not effective that self-inflicted injury will be confirmed. This approach is helpful by offering the patient the choice of either stopping interfering with the wound or accepting the opportunity to receive psychotherapy. It also avoids the patient transferring to another healthcare professional for the cycle to be repeated.

Management

The long-term outcome for these young patients is poor, with 30% of wounds staying unhealed in the long term (Sneddon and Sneddon 1975).

This is undoubtedly a very difficult aspect of care to manage. Accurate documentation of the patient and wound assessment is crucial. The experienced nurse may well be able to identify the situation where the appearance of the wound and the history the patient gives do not correspond. The first line of management should be to exclude physical causes for non-healing, which are often difficult to detect, and to obtain as much information as possible from previous medical and nursing notes. Remember that the patient may have received treatment in other hospitals or other parts of the country. Systemic and local infections need to be promptly treated as serious illness could result from such infection. Precautions against infections spread by blood and body fluids should be strictly adhered to as there is a risk of hepatitis and HIV infection.

Above all, the nurse's manner and approach to the young individual in these difficult circumstances need careful thought. It is important for the nurse not to judge the patient by his or her own standards and to appreciate the complex nature of factitious illness.

The use of dressings which require infrequent dressing changes with the minimum of fuss take the focus away from the wound. Occlusive dressings, such as hydrocolloids, also prevent the transmission of bacteria from the environment to the wound bed and help prevent the patient interfering with the wound.

Nursing model for Justina

Look back over this young woman's history: what do you suspect may be the cause of her wound?

The obvious conclusion would be that she is an injecting drug abuser and has used her leg veins for access; but unless Justina is prepared to give Sister Andrews this information, how can it be proved?

The important feature of this case will be the nurse–patient interaction, therefore Sister Andrews can use the Riehl interaction model (Riehl 1980). The key information to be collected is the patient's 'definition' of the situation, therefore the nurse must attempt to enter into the patient's world in order to understand her viewpoint. Riehl underplays the physiological systems as the determinants of patients' problems, emphasizing the importance of psychosocial aspects.

In the first stage of the assessment it is necessary to ascertain if Justina is adopting an appropriate role for her situation.

- Assessment (Stage 1): is Justina adopting an appropriate role for her present situation? (no)
- Planning (Stage 2): what are her problems related to?
    physical?   (yes)
    psychological?   (yes)
    sociological?   (yes)

It is necessary to identify the problems (Table 6.4) and negotiate patient-centred goals (Table 6.5).

Table 6.4 *Identification of Justina's problems (Case Study 6.5)*

Psychological	Physical	Sociological
Denial of cause of wound (A)	Necrotic non-healing wound (A)	Involved in drug taking subculture (A)
Barrier between nurse and patient (A)	Localized infection (A)	Not in long-term employment (A)
Requires help for wound but reluctant to seek it (A)	Invasive infection and septicaemia (P)	Lives in squalid housing conditions (A)
Stigma associated with type of wound (A)	Loss of use of foot/limb (P)	
Fear of drug problem being exposed (A)	Infection with HIV, AIDS (A or P) Addition to abusive substance (A)	

(A), actual problem; (P), potential problem.

Table 6.5 *Patient-centred goals and interventions planned for Justina (Case Study 6.5)*

Goal	Intervention
Psychological Enable patient to reveal her problem of drug abuse by forming a trusting relationship between nurse and patient	i) Display a non-judgemental attitude to Justina when attending to the wound ii) Give ample opportunity for Justina to discuss her problems iii) Stress confidentiality of treatment and any patient details recorded iv) Ensure treatment time will be undisturbed by other members of the practice v) Indicate that you are aware of her problem, but will only discuss it if she wishes vi) Allow Justina to see her records — do not hide them from her
To form a trusting relationship between nurse and patient	i) Display a concerned attitude towards Justina's general physical and mental condition ii) Involve Justina in planning care for her wound, and seek her opinion iii) Explain the nature of wound healing and the risk of possible infection iv) Ensure Justina knows whom to contact if the condition of the wound deteriorates v) Encourage Justina to discuss her relationship with family and friends vi) Ensure that she is given correct information regarding the treatment plan
Physiological Removal of necrotic tissue to promote healing of wound	i) Cover wound with a hydrocolloid dressing to promote autolysis and provide a protective barrier ii) Take a wound swab to confirm the type of organisms present in the wound iii) Teach Justina safe methods of cleaning her wound and reapplying the dressing (role play) iv) Liaise with community nurses to arrange home visits v) Document size, site and appearance of wound on initial and subsequent visits
To prevent spread of infection systemically	i) Explain the importance of keeping the wound clean ii) Ensure use of gloves when removing and reapplying dressings iii) Doctor to prescribe course of prophylactic antibiotics iv) Explain importance of taking antibiotic cover v) Arrange a mutually convenient time for Justina to attend the surgery
Sociological To facilitate opportunities for Justina to improve her socio-economic status	i) Provide information regarding helplines, drug counsellors, etc. ii) Ensure Justina has appropriate benefit entitlement

Practice points

- Justina belongs to a subculture where drug taking is the norm and personal self-esteem is low.

- Sister Andrews attempts to build a relationship with Justina by involving her in her care and seeking her opinion.

- She realizes that Justina may not attend the surgery again, so attempts to teach her some kind of self-care, but also liaises with the community nurses. Much of her care is a form of role play because she demonstrates to Justina that she is non-judgemental about her drug abuse but cares about her physical condition.

- She cannot cure the drug problem but she provides opportunities for Justina to seek help if desired.

- The wound may not heal, especially if Justina tries to gain access to a vein in the same site.

- The overall aim of management, therefore, is not necessarily wound healing but to gain the patient's trust so that her real problem (drug abuse) can be dealt with.

Summary

This chapter has reflected on five different examples of the range of situations encountered by young adults.

Mostly healing will take place in this age group without too many physiological complications; however, psychological and sociological problems will require as much if not more attention to ensure the patient reaches a satisfactory outcome.

The type of models used highlight the following important issues:

- the patient and nurse plan care together to meet the patient's needs
- the nurse can attempt to understand the problems from the patient's perspective
- the effect the wound will have on the normal living patterns of the patient
- the range of dressings available that the patient can manage alone
- the nurse remains non-judgemental and uses her counselling skills to gain the patient's trust

These are skills that are gained through clinical experience and reflective practice.

Look for somebody in your clinical area who you feel possesses these skills, and watch how they interact with their patients.

Further Reading   Mishtriki SK, Jeffery PJ & Law DJW (1992) Wound infection: the surgeon's responsibility. *Journal of Wound Care* 1(2): 32–36.

Eagle M (1993) The care of a patient after a caesarean section. *Journal of Wound Care* 2(6): 330–336.

Harkiss KJ (ed.) (1970) *Surgical Dressings and Wound Healing*. Bradford University Press.

Müller C, O'Neill A & Mortimer D (1993) Skin problems in palliative care: nursing aspects. In: Doyle D, Hanks G & McDonald N (eds) *Oxford Textbook in Palliative Medicine*. Oxford: Oxford Medical.

Grocott P (1995) The palliative management of fungating malignant wounds. *Journal of Wound Care* 4(5): 240–242.

McConnel EA (1991) Surgical patient care. In: *Illustrated Manual of Nursing Practice*. Springhouse Penn: Springhouse.

Dealey C (1994) *The care of wounds*. Oxford. Blackwell.

References   Baragwanath P, Shutler S & Harding KG (1994a) The management of a patient with a factitious wound. *Journal of Wound Care* 3(6): 286–287.

Baragwanath P, Gruffudd-Jones A, Young HL & Harding KG (1994b) Factitious behaviour in the aetiology of non-healing wounds. *Proceedings of the Fourth European Conference on Advances in Wound Management* London: Macmillan.

Berry DP (1992) Pilonidal sinus disease. *Journal of Wound Care* 1(3): 29–32.

Buie LA & Curtis PD (1952) Pilonidal disease. *Surgical Clinics of North America* 32: 1247–1259.

Clothier PR & Haywood IR (1984) The natural history of postnasal (pilonidal) sinus. *Annals of the Royal College of Surgeons* 66: 201–203.

Department of Health (1991) *The Patients' Charter*. London: HMSO.

Drinker H, Knorr N & Edgerton M (1972) Factitious wounds: a psychiatric and surgical dilemma. *Plastic and Reconstructive Surgery* 50: 458–461.

Eisedrath S (1989) Factitious physical disorders: treatment without confrontation. *Psychosomatics* 30: 383–387.

Fras I & Coughlin B (1972) The treatment of factitial disease. *Psychosomatics* 12: 117–122.

Harrison BJ, Read GF & Hughes LE (1988) Endocrine basis for the clinical presentation of hidradenitis suppurativa. *British Journal of Surgery* 75: 972–975.

Jones DJ (1992) Pilonidal sinus. *British Medical Journal* 305: 410–412.

Lyell A (1972) Dermatitis artefacta and self-inflicted disease. *Scottish Medical Journal* 17: 187–196.

Macleod J, Edwards C & Bouchier I (1987) Diseases of connective tissues, joint and bones. In: *Davidson's Principles and Practices of Medicine*, Chapter 14. Edinburgh: Churchill Livingstone.

Orem D (1980) *Nursing – Concepts of Practice*. New York: McGraw Hill.

Peplau H (1952) *Interpersonal Relations in Nursing*. New York: Putman.

Riehl JP (1980) The Riehl interaction model. In: Riehl JP & Roy C (eds) *Conceptual Models for Nursing Practice*. New York: Appleton-Century-Crofts.

Rodgers SE (1994) The patient facing surgery. In: *Nursing Practice* p. 775. Alexander MF, Fawcett JN & Rucerian PJ (eds) Edinburgh: Churchill Livingstone.

Roy C (1980) The Roy adaptation model. In: Riehl JP & Roy C (eds) *Conceptual Models for Nursing Practice*. New York: Appleton-Century-Crofts.

Smitherman C (1981) *Nursing Actions for Health Promotion*. Philadelphia: Davis.

Sneddon I & Sneddon J (1975) Self-inflicted injury: a follow-up study of 43 patients. *British Medical Journal* 3: 527–530.

Wood RAB, Williams RHP & Hughes LE (1972) Foam elastomer dressing in the management of open granulating wounds: experience with 250 patients. *British Journal of Surgery* 64: 554–557.

7 Wound Care in the Middle-aged Individual

Key issues

This chapter outlines the wound problems encountered by the middle-aged individual.

Clinical Case Studies

Aetiology and management of the following:

- Neuropathic foot ulcer in a man with diabetes mellitus
- Postoperative care of a patient following a partial mastectomy and breast reconstruction
- A patient undergoing abdominal perineal resection

Nursing Models

Examples of their application to practice are taken from:

- Peplau's model
- Roy's adaptation model
- Orem's model

Practice points

- As you read through this chapter concentrate on the following:
- the effect of serious illness on a previously healthy adult
- the nurse in an educative and supportive role
- the use of specialist nurses to complement the care given to these patients
- the importance that underlying disease processes have on wound healing

Introduction

For many individuals the teenage and adult years are full of activity, parenting and hard work. Middle age can bring financial stability and contentment. When illness happens at this stage of the life-cycle patients can have difficulty accepting it. Malignancy, diabetes mellitus and cardiovascular disease are frequently encountered diseases for this age group.

Diabetic Foot Ulceration

Diabetic foot ulcers are a serious complication of diabetes mellitus. The problem can be compounded by the patient's lifestyle, as in Case Study 7.1.

Case Study 7.1
Diabetic foot ulceration

Donald Waites has had insulin-dependent diabetes mellitus for 30 years, having been diagnosed at the age of 25 years. Following diagnosis of his condition Donald was very careful in following the advice given and took his insulin according to his blood glucose levels. Patient education was sparse at that time as there were no specialist nurses or clinics and management was largely controlled by the hospital consultant or general practitioner. As time progressed, like many individuals with diabetes mellitus, Donald began to disregard advice and gave himself extra insulin when going out for a large meal and drinking heavily.

In his 30s and 40s he had many epsiodes of hypoglycaemia and hyperglycaemia, which on several occasions resulted in admission to hospital. Education regarding diet, weight control and foot care was reinforced on these occasions but by now Donald was becoming resistant to the advice of health professionals, feeling that he had received little support in coping with his condition over the years. These periods of hospitalization resulted in Donald's employment becoming sporadic, and he often found himself without work and having to claim unemployment benefit in order to support himself.

At present Donald, now 55 years old, is working on a building site as a bricklayer. He is single and has no dependants. Working long hours to claim overtime, he continues to bypass regular meals or insulin. His personal hygiene has also deteriorated and his housing conditions are squalid.

As far as diabetic management goes, he has not visited his general practitioner for the last 2 years, even though he has been experiencing 'pins and needles' in his arms and hands and a loss of sensation in both feet. This has frightened Donald as at this time of his life he is fearful of not having employment and being unable to draw a pension.

On return from work yesterday Donald took off his boot and found he had a round ulcer on his right heel. The skin surrounding the wound was red and inflamed, and although he could feel nothing he realized it had been caused by a nail sticking through the heel of his boot. Donald remembered a patient in the bed next to him during his last hospital visit who had had a similar ulcer, and also remembered that this man ended up having his leg amputated. Donald went to his doctor the very next morning.

Aetiology

Diabetic foot problems are the cause of more inpatient stays than all the other medical problems caused by diabetes (Tunbridge and Hare 1990). The impact of foot ulceration on the individual's life is great, with the potential for amputation ever-present. Williams (1994) has estimated that in the UK there are around 750 000 patients with diabetes mellitus. Of this group, 4% will have had an amputation, with a further 6% experiencing foot ulceration. This translates into around 30 000 patients either missing a limb or part of a limb, and 45 000 patients currently having foot ulceration. The two main causes of foot ulceration for diabetic patients are peripheral neuropathy and peripheral vascular disease — with the presence of infection exacerbating the problem considerably. Both peripheral neuropathy and peripheral vascular disease can occur simultaneously, and where infection is present this can lead to soft tissue necrosis and possibly damage to underlying tendon and bone. The prevalence of both neuropathy and peripheral vascular disease increases with the duration of the diabetic condition. Below the age of 40 years foot ulceration is uncommon. Around 6% of diabetic patients aged 60–69 years experience foot ulceration, rising to 14% in those patients aged 80 years and over (Walters *et al.* 1992). The nerve damage caused by diabetic neuropathy is generally thought to be the result of the accumulation of metabolites of glucose, which causes osmotic swelling and damage to nerve cells (McIntyre 1994).

■ Peripheral neuropathy — neuropathic ulcers are by far the most common cause of diabetic foot ulceration and are a serious complication of diabetes (Figure 7.1). Most commonly peripheral neuropathy affects the lower limbs, and can affect either sensory, motor or cutaneous nerves. Sensory impairment means that painless neuropathic ulcers can be caused by repeated pressure and trauma from ill-fitting shoes. Thermal trauma may be caused by the heat of fires or hot-water bottles, which the patient fails

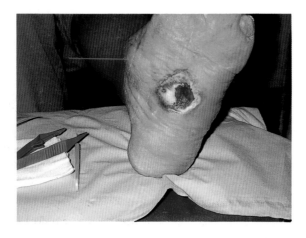

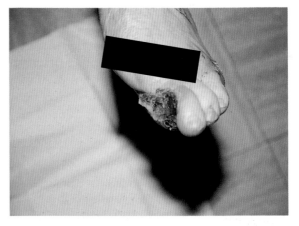

Figure 7.1 *A neuropathic foot ulcer showing Charcot's joints of the foot.*

Figure 7.2 *Patient with peripheral vascular disease due to diabetes. The great and first toe have already been amputated due to gangrene.*

to feel. Chemical trauma may result from the diabetic patient applying home remedies, such as over-the-counter treatment for corns, instead of consulting a chiropodist. Patients with neuropathy may cut their toenails too harshly, get sunburnt feet, or step on a sharp object without realizing that damage is being done.

Ischaemia
the deficiency in blood supply to a part of the body due to functional constriction or actual obstruction of a blood vessel

■ Peripheral vascular disease — vascular insufficiency affects, in the first instance, the smaller arterioles of the lower limbs. The distal cells are deprived of the necessary metabolic requirements and the tissues become devitalized. Subsequent injury from ill-fitting footwear can then readily cause **ischaemic** ulceration of the area (Figure 7.2).

Thrombosis can also occur, resulting in gangrene of the area supplied by the thrombosed vessel. So, gangrene can result from a seemingly minor injury, with very serious consequences. Both life and limb are at risk in this situation. The affected limb, or part of the limb, may require amputation, with infection and septicaemia being potentially lethal.

Identifying the patient at risk of developing foot ulceration is essential if ulceration is to be prevented or damage minimized. Connor (1994) has identified risk factors for diabetic patients (Table 7.1).

Many diabetic foot problems can be prevented or the damage minimized through careful monitoring of the patient's feet. Protective measures are listed in Table 7.2.

Table 7.1   *Risk factors for developing ulceration or gangrene*

1. Previous ulceration or gangrene
2. Increasing age
3. Peripheral vascular disease
4. Neuropathy
5. Structural deformity
6. The feckless patient
7. Other:
   duration of diabetes
   male sex
   retinopathy
   nephropathy
   living alone

From Connor (1994).

Assessment and Diagnosis

A full history and examination should be performed relating to the patient's diabetes. If this has already been done, accurate documentation should be obtained of the previous history.

Central to the diagnosis is an integrated clinical examination of the foot (Figure 7.3). Assessment should aim to:

Table 7.2   *Measures to protect the feet in diabetes mellitus*

General measures
Do not smoke
Take a healthy diet with lots of fibre and not too much fat
Try to keep body weight within normal limits
Exercise. Try to keep active. This will help the circulation
Get blood pressure and blood fats checked regularly

Footwear
Try to get shoes which don't pinch anywhere and which allow all toes to move freely. Break in new shoes very gradually
Ensure that socks or stockings fit comfortably. Change them daily
Change footwear as soon as possible if wet
Avoid walking barefoot; wear slippers and beach shoes to prevent injury

Foot care
Bathe feet daily using lukewarm (not hot) water and soap
Pat feet dry gently; pay special attention to the area between the toes
Apply a lanolin-based moisturizing cream daily to avoid dryness and keep the skin supple
Avoid exposing feet to excess heat or cold
Avoid sunburn to the feet and legs
Cut nails straight across while they are still soft from bathing
Inspect feet daily for blisters, corns, calluses, cracks or redness (a mirror can help in seeing the underside of the foot)
If a minor cut or abrasion does occur, wash thoroughly and cover with a clean dressing. See your doctor if the cut has not healed in 48 hours
Your chiropodist should be consulted for treatment of ingrown toenails, corns, calluses or verrucae (no home remedies, please)
A doctor or nurse should be consulted if foot problems such as tingling, numbness, swelling, pain or loss of feeling develop
Remember: most people with diabetes never have any trouble with their feet. Take reasonable care of your feet and they will reward you by lasting a lifetime!

From Fawcett *et al.* (1994).

Figure 7.3
Neuropathic ulcers of both feet. These wounds require debridement of necrotic tissue and callus before wound assessment can take place.

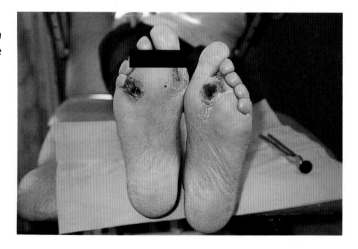

- Ascertain the type, onset and duration of diabetes
- Identify current or developing complications of diabetes
- Diagnose the exact nature and aetiology of the ulcer
- Prescribe the correct medical or surgical treatment
- Identify suitable dressing and foot care that will enhance healing

Important points to be recorded are summarized in Table 7.3, while Table 7.4 lists the clinical features that differentiate neuropathic and ischaemic ulceration.

Table 7.3 *Important facts to be ascertained in patients with diabetic ulceration*

Record	Rationale
Date of birth	Age is a risk factor for PVD
Sex	PVD and amputations more common in men
Type of diabetes and treatment	Methods of achieving good control. May change treatment if control poor
Duration of diabetes	Prevalence of neuropathy and ischaemia increase with duration
History of ischaemic heart disease, myocardial infarctions, cerebrovascular accident, angina	Indication of arteriosclerosis and ischaemia
Smoking	Risk factor for PVD in diabetic patients
Compliance	Key factor in aetiology of ulcer and after-care management
History of intermittent claudication	Indicative of ischaemia
Rest pain	
Previous arterial surgery	

PVD, peripheral vascular disease.

Specific examinations

For ischaemia

Doppler assessment and measurement of ankle brachial pressure index (see Chapter 9) will indicate an ischaemic cause for the ulceration. The Doppler ultrasound reading can be used in conjunction with clinical examination to confirm the presence of ischaemia. Patients with diabetes mellitus may give falsely high (i.e. normal) readings owing to calcification of the arteries.

For neuropathy

The vibration threshold is measured using a biothesiometer; vibrations can be transmitted through the patient's foot to indicate the extent of sensory loss.

Other examinations

Retinal examination indicates the absence or degree of retinopathy. Other investigations are listed in Table 7.5.

Table 7.4   *Differential diagnosis of neuropathic and ischaemic ulceration*

Clinical feature	Neuropathic foot	Ischaemic foot
Colour	Normal or red appearance indicating cellulitis or early Charcot foot	Pale/cyanotic Rubor on dependency Blanches on elevation (Buerger's test)
Deformity	Claw toe Hammer toe Charcot deformity	Nil Absent toes from previous surgery
Callus tissue	Found on plantar surface of metatarsal head/apices or toes	Nil — thin skin
Tissue breakdown	Ulcers commonly found on plantar surface	Ulcers commonly found on the margins Visible signs of digital gangrene
Peripheral pulses	Present (may be difficult to palpate if swollen or deformed foot)	Dorsalis pedis and/or posterior tibial absent May not be absent if small vessel disease
Temperature	Feels normal or warm	Feels cold
Skin moisture	Dry foot Decrease in perspiration	Normal
Sensation	Impaired sensation to pinprick/light touch position and vibration	Normal
Tendon reflex	Impaired	Normal

From Wound Healing Research Unit (1994).

Table 7.5   *Other investigations in diabetic foot ulceration*

Record	Rationale
Haemoglobin HbA, C	Good measure of long-term control
Urea and creatinine	Measurement of renal function indicative of nephropathy
Proteinuria	Indicative of nephropathy
Wound swab	Confirms clinical signs of infection

Management

Healing is likely to be impaired in the patient with diabetes mellitus as there is a reduction in the inflammatory response and granulation tissue formation. Neuropathic ulcers usually take weeks or months to heal, even with the appropriate resources. Some patients require complete bed rest combined with removal of weight-bearing and friction. For patients with ischaemic ulcers, reconstructive arterial surgery may be required, though healing can be achieved in 60% of these patients with good medical management (Foster 1987). For patients with ulceration of both types an overall healing rate of 63% has been achieved (Abelqvist 1990).

- General issues related to the disease process of diabetes mellitus should be considered, i.e. control of the disease and referral to the appropriate specialist for reconstructive surgery or medical treatment of complications.

- Continuing care and maintenance of the foot can be given, ideally at a multidisciplinary foot clinic, or by a chiropodist. Nail and foot care can be provided and problems detected at an early stage.

- Ideally all weight should be relieved from the ulcerated area and redistributed. This can be achieved by an orthotist designing and making footwear for the patient.

- Daily inspection of the feet by the patient should be undertaken, regardless of whether the foot is ulcerated or not. Any signs of redness, heat, blistering or bleeding should be looked for and immediate treatment sought. If ignored, the foot could rapidly deteriorate and lead to invasive infection of the limb.

- Dressings useful for the treatment of foot ulceration include absorbent foams which act as padding and protection for the injured area. For moderate or heavily exuding ulcers alginate dressings can provide absorbency without too much bulk. Occlusive dressings such as hydrocolloids or adhesive dressings which are not changed daily and so prevent daily foot inspection are best avoided.

- Regular debridement of callus build-up around the ulcer bed is advised. All callus, or as much as possible, should be removed to prevent further trauma to the area.

Nursing model for Donald

Having visited his general practitioner, who performed a full assessment (see below), Donald was diagnosed as having a neuropathic foot ulcer.

The general practitioner transferred wound care to the district nurse. If the district nurse uses Peplau's model to assess and plan Donald's care, what particular aspects of the model are pertinent to this patient's care?

Development models often focus on the educative-counselling role the nurse plays. This has paramount importance, as often the care a patient needs may be different from what he or she wants. Do you think that Donald wants the care and advice the district nurse is going to give? (Probably he does not.)

Peplau's philosophy of nursing stresses the importance of the formation of the relationship between nurse and patient. The first purpose of the nurse is to minimize or remove the risks to the patient's health, but the second is to help the individual to understand and come to terms with their health problem. In Donald's case this will require a great deal of input.

Look at Tables 7.6 and 7.7, compiled using the SOAP acronym (S, subjective experience of patient; O, objective observation made by nurse; A, assessment and identification of problems on S and O; P, plan of action).

Practice point

- Donald Waites' case stresses the importance of the nurse's role in helping patients to understand and come to terms with their condition.

Table 7.6   *Assessment of Donald's problems (Case Study 7.1)*

Subjective experience of patient	Objective observation by nurse
Little faith in health professionals	Patient non-compliant with treatment
Not wanting to be labelled as ill	Patient unaware of health status
Feels he can control illness by altering insulin according to social needs	Little understanding of the pathology of the disease process
Frightened of the consequences of his complaint	Has not reported signs of neuropathy until ulcer developed Displaying signs of advanced disease process
Frightened that ulceration could lead to amputation	Localized infection in and around ulcer, possibility of invasive infection
Does not understand why he did not feel nail in shoe rubbing	Not aware of signs of diabetic neuropathy Does not inspect feet daily
Finds it increasingly difficult to keep up with personal hygiene and domestic chores	Looks unkempt; nobody at home to provide support
Worried that period of sickness will result in unemployment	Financial difficulties due to sporadic employment

Table 7.7   *Identification of problems in Table 7.6 and plan of action*

Identification of problem	Plan of action
Infected neuropathic ulcer	Debridement of ulcer by doctor, nurse or chiropodist Daily dressing with absorbent dressing (foam or alginate), wound cleansing with saline to remove dressing material Swab to identify infecting organism, treat with broad-spectrum antibiotic orally initially One-week period of non-weight bearing
Poor understanding of diet and diabetic control	Diabetic specialist nurse and community dietician to visit patient at home District nurse to reinforce information with patient education programme
Long-term history of unstable diabetes	Assessment of HbAc blood test Renal function, eye retinopathy, extent of neuropathy Referral to diabetic specialist
Lack of knowledge concerning care of feet	District nurse to explain importance of inspection of feet daily, hygiene and clean footwear Refer to orthotist for removal of friction Refer to chiropodist
Reluctant to seek support of health professionals	District nurse to promote a trusting relationship with patient by listening to his point of view Planning care together with realistic goals Introducing other specialists to patient at separate intervals
Lives alone, no social support	Encourage patient to joint local diabetic association; find out details of local group
Fear of loss of employment and lack of secure income	Arrange visit of social worker to reassess benefit entitlement Consider change of employment to less manual work

Breast Cancer

Case Study 7.2 outlines the case of a woman who has undergone a partial mastectomy for removal of a breast tumour.

Case Study 7.2 Partial mastectomy and breast reconstruction	Mrs Joyce Harris is recovering in hospital following a partial mastectomy and breast reconstruction. The operation to remove a tumour from her left breast was performed 4 days ago. She now has two transverse suture lines, one across the reconstructed left breast, the other across her abdomen from which tissue was taken to perform the reconstructive surgery.
	Joyce, who is 46 years old, is progressing well and is pleased with the cosmetic results of her breast. She has been informed that all the tumour was removed and does not require any further treatment.
	The suture lines are clean and non-inflamed.

Aetiology

In the UK around 15 000 women die as a result of breast cancer, with it being the most common form of cancer affecting women (Parker 1994). Breast cancer is rare under the age of 35 years, but the incidence increases with age with most women being diagnosed between 45 years and 75 years of age. A family history of a close relative with cancer also increases the risk.

Around 75% of breast cancers are ductal cancers originating from the epithelial cells of the breast ducts, and are commonly confined to one area of the breast. Around 15% of breast cancers are lobular carcinomas originating from the cells of the breast lobules. These are more likely to be multifocal and bilateral. The extent or severity of the cancer is classified as follows:

- non-invasive — the malignant cells are contained with the originating tissue and have not spread outwards into surrounding tissues, the cancer remains in situ within the tissue of origin.

- invasive — the malignant cells have spread into the surrounding tissues.

- differentiation — the malignant cells are histologically described as being poorly, moderately or well differentiated. Well-differentiated malignant cells closely resemble the tissue in which they originated. They are less aggressive than poorly differentiated cells, which metastasize (spread to distant sites) at an early stage.

Diagnosis

Following the discovery of a lump or mass in the breast or detection of a mass on mammography, the woman should be encouraged to attend her general practitioner for referral to a breast specialist centre. It is likely that a number of investigations will be performed at this early stage. A full medical history will be taken by the breast specialist, followed by a physical examination including clinical examination of the breast. The woman will almost certainy be extremely anxious and concerned about her well-being and would be best advised for this crucial hospital visit to be accompanied by her partner or a friend. Other investigations carried out at this time include a mammogram, fine-needle aspiration of the mass or lump for cytology, ultrasonography to differentiate between lumps and cysts, and biopsy. It will take several days for the results of these types of investigation to be reported and for the breast specialist to make a firm diagnosis. This is an extremely stressful time for the woman and her family. The choice of treatment offered depends on several factors (Parker 1994).

- The size, position and type of tumour
- The spread of the disease
- The woman's general health
- The wishes of the individual woman

Surgery, radiotherapy or chemotherapy may be offered. Surgery may range from a simple excision of the breast lump to a wide local excision of the lump, partial or segmental mastectomy, or simple mastectomy possibly with axillary dissection of lymph glands. Radiotherapy and chemotherapy may be offered in addition to surgery. All postmenopausal women are offered an oestrogen blocking drug, tamoxifen, as an adjuvant therapy. Postmenopausal women have high levels of oestrogen receptors and this drug works by blocking the oestrogen from stimulating cancer cell growth.

Despite the advances in treatment of breast cancer it has not been possible to reduce the mortality rate for this disease. The earlier women are diagnosed the greater the chance for survival. Overall, only 64% of women with breast cancer will be alive 5 years later. When diagnosed in the early stage 84% of women will survive to 5 years, the message being that the earlier breast cancer is detected the better the prognosis.

Post-operative Care

The suture lines need to be observed for the signs of clinical infection and this observation linked to measurements of temperature and pulse. The primary wound dressing can be left undisturbed if a transparent dressing has been used and only changed if it becomes too soiled. It is also usual for low-suction drainage to be used; one drain is inserted under the suture lines and another in the axillary area, both sites where haematoma formation is likely. After 48 hours these may be removed when the drainage subsides.

Nursing model for Joyce

Joyce requires basic post-operative care for her wounds. The surgery has been elective and at a site with a low risk of contamination. However, think of the wider implications of this type of surgery and the cosmetic and psychological effects this type of wound has on any woman.

Joyce needs to adapt to her new body image and the loss of what she may feel as sexual attractiveness; maybe Roy's adaptation model would be a good choice here (Table 7.8).

Table 7.8   *Application of Roy's assessment model to the problems of Mrs Harris (Case Study 7.2)*

Life Area	Assessment Level 1 — Behaviour	Assessment Level 2 — Stimuli		
		Focal	**Contextual**	**Residual**
Physiological Rest and activity	Unable to move arm and sit up straight	Wound painful		Fear of splitting stitches
Regulation	Pain in breast and abdomen	Surgery, anxiety	Afraid to bother nurses for pain relief	Afraid to take too many pain-killers
	Wound dehiscence Wound infection	No obvious signs	Wound breakdown likely at 10 days	
Self-concept	Worried about scarring	Wound sutured	Underlying malignancy may retard healing	Has heard bad reports of breast reconstruction
	Loss of 'normal' body appearance	Left breast shape different from right	Final shape may differ	Breast shape not as shown in pictures of reconstruction
	Fear of recurrence of disease	Only lump removed, not whole breast	Doctors cannot give 100% assurance	Has no experience of others with same problem
Role function	Loss of femininity	Sutured wounds ugly	Feels tired and depressed after operation	
	Loss of role as husband's sexual partner	Husband's anxiety has changed his manner with her		

Practice points

- By assessing the focal, contextual or residual origins of the various problems, the nurse can plan appropriate interventions.

- What are the major features required to give Joyce optimum care? Wound care may not be the most important issue in this case. The services of the specialist breast nurse should be enlisted to provide support and advice to this patient.

Colorectal Cancer

Case Study 7.3 illustrates the problems that may follow an abdominoperineal resection for colorectal cancer.

Case Study 7.3 Abdomino-perineal resection

Harold Mathews is a 62-year-old man, a widower for 10 years, who runs a large dairy farm with his two sons.

He had, for some time, experienced problems with a change in his bowel habit and eventually was persuaded by his elder son to go and see his doctor.

Harold was admitted to hospital for tests and diagnosed as having an adenocarcinoma of the rectum. An abdominoperineal resection was performed within a matter of days following diagnosis, leaving Harold with a colostomy, a sutured laparotomy line and a perineal wound left open to heal by secondary intention. Harold was determined to recover quickly as he was not used to hospital and disliked people fussing over him.

Preoperatively Harold was visited by the stoma therapist who helped him decide where to site his stoma and which appliances to use. During the post-operative period Harold quickly mastered changing the colostomy bags and gained confidence. His laparotomy wound healed well and sutures were removed 10 days post-operatively.

Harold's perineal wound measured 6 cm long, 3 cm wide and 8 cm deep on discharge from hospital. Granulation tissue had covered the wound bed which was healthy and clean. In hospital the wound had been irrigated daily while the patient was taking a shower and the ward nurses had taken considerable care to treat this as part of his daily hygiene. Once Harold had dried after showering an absorbent pad protected his clean pyjamas until he returned to his bed for a dressing renewal. The perineal wound was inspected carefully at these daily dressing changes, the nurses looking for pocketing and tracking in the depths of the wound, and wound measurements were taken weekly. The wound was packed with an alginate rope which Harold found comfortable and absorbent.

He was discharged home after 10 days in hospital, to the care of the district nurse who would look after his perineal wound on a daily basis using alginate and monitor his progress. On his first evening home Harold appeared to lose all confidence and panicked. His younger son, who still lives on the farm, found him in the early hours of the morning in the bathroom crying because his stoma bag had come loose during the night and had soiled his pyjamas. The district nurse was due to call that day.

Aetiology

Colorectal cancer in the Western world is the second largest cause of death from cancers, most commonly occurring in people over 40 years old. Cancer of the rectum and sigmoid colon is most common, with men mostly affected with rectal carcinoma and women with colonic carcinoma (Miller *et al.* 1994). The cause of colorectal cancer is difficult to determine, but it has been linked to the low-residue diet and lifestyle of the affluent populations (Burkitt 1971).

The onset of the disease is often gradual and it is not unusual for patients to present to their general practitioner only when the disease is at an advanced stage. Patients experience vague symptoms of a gradual change of bowel habit, with constipation alternating with diarrhoea.

Management

Middle-aged and elderly individuals are often reluctant to present to their doctor with symptoms related to colorectal disease. Very often the onset of colorectal cancer is gradual and vague, often without pain until the cancer obstructs or partially obstructs the colon. Patients can easily mistake bleeding and mucus in the stool for haemorrhoids, with changes in bowel habit being related to problems with food. It is common for patients to present with bowel obstruction and acute abdominal pain. Emergency surgery is likely to result in the tumour being excised together with the rectum and the formation of a permanent colostomy. There can be little time to prepare the patient for this extensive, disfiguring surgery. Around 100 000 people in the UK have a stoma of some type, be that colostomy, ileostomy or urostomy. Of these, some 30 000 have a permanent colostomy and around 6500 patients a year have a permanent colostomy formed (Liles 1995). Many patients experience extreme trauma following formation of a permanent colostomy. Body image is severely altered, leading to anxiety, loss of confidence, rejection, social isolation, depression and sexual dysfunction. Patients can feel that the surgery has mutilated their body (Kelly 1985). Patients with a colostomy can find that their lifestyle is changed beyond recognition in the initial months following surgery, owing to the loss of control of their bowel habits and the struggle to gain control of the stoma (Willis 1995).

The help of a specialist stoma nurse pre-operatively where possible and also in the post-operative period is invaluable in providing both counselling and practical help and advice. Patients should have the opportunity to choose the stoma appliance most suited to their lifestyle. This is a stressful time for patients: having to accept a permanent stoma is difficult when recovering from unexpected major surgery.

Deep perineal wounds require careful observation and dressing. Assessments and measurements weekly should demonstrate steady progress towards healing, with evidence that the wound is healing from its depths with reduction in both depth and width as wound contraction takes place. Gentle examination of the wound should exclude pocketing and premature bridging in the depths of the wound. The professional help and support

Table 7.9 *Self-care deficits for Harold Mathews (Case Study 7.3)*

Normal self-care ability (prior to operation)	Current self-care ability (following discharge home)	Self-care deficit (lack of knowledge, skill, motivation or limited behaviour)
Fluid balance Likes to drink beer (usually 2–3 pints at the weekend) Drinks large quantities of tea while working on farm	Rather dehydrated following operation, felt nauseous for some days, finds he does not have a 'taste' for drinks	
Nutrition Eats cooked breakfast and large cooked evening meal Lots of meat and vegetables	Loss of weight due to disease Does not feel like eating and worried about effect on colostomy	
Activity and rest Up at 5.30 every morning, works most of day until 8 at night Always active	Weak following surgery Wants to do things but cannot, feels frustrated and angry	
Socialization Lives with son since wife died 10 years ago. Eats together with other son and daughter-in-law every Sunday Socializes in pub at weekends, at church on Sunday	Depressed and embarrassed about colostomy Worried he will smell when in church or having lunch Does not want sons to know about the bag	
Hazards Worries that once his son leaves he will be unable to manage farm and farmhouse	Worried about sons coping without him Long-term worries about how he will manage if son goes, now he has been so ill	
Normalcy Misses his wife greatly, as she helped on the farm as well as in the house	Has no-one to confide in and care for him Has managed to cope since his wife died, but feels out of control Does not want a nurse coming to the farm	
Health previously Never had reason to go to doctor Always uses local remedy to treat himself	Worried about the care of an open wound on farm Feels invalided and old Feels surgery was drastic and disease could have taken its course Does not know if he can resume normal work pattern	

initiated in hospital in the immediate post-operative phase will need to be continued once the patient has returned home.

Nursing model for Harold

Think about the type of person Harold is before planning his care. A farmer all his life, still very active in the running of his farm, he is used to looking after himself since widowed.

He needs a long period of recuperation and support from those providing care, but probably needs to regain as much independence as possible. It often happens that patients in hospital feel confident and appear on the surface to be coming to terms with their surgery. A large operation such as this requires long-term management.

Using Orem's model, we can assess Harold's deficits. The district nurse should, of course, decide whether these deficits are due to lack of knowledge, skill, motivation or limited range of behaviour (Table 7.9). Can you identify his self-care deficits?

Practice points

This type of situation is not uncommon. Patients often feel alone and fearful following discharge from the security of the hospital.

- The district nurse will need to gain Harold's confidence but also should enlist the support of specialist nurses and other primary care team members to help him recover a normal social pattern.

- His feelings are similar to those experienced when he lost his wife, and the nurse must be aware of this.

- A plan of care *must* take into account his previous pattern of work on the farm as much as possible. This should include minimum dressing changes, using one that will remain in situ.

Summary

Throughout this chapter there are two fundamental aspects that need to be addressed in order to provide a high level of wound care for an individual in this age group. They are:

■ the transition from health to *serious* illness in an adult requires the nurse to function in an educative role

■ all these cases require the input of specialist nurses who with their expert skills give a high level of professional care to their patients.

If you work with any specialist practitioners, observe the skills they use to enhance patient care.

Further Reading

Elkeles RS & Wolfe JHN (1993) The diabetic foot. ABC of vascular disease. *British Medical Journal* 303: 1053–1055.

Foster A (1987) Examination of the diabetic foot: Part II. *Practical Diabetes* 4(4): 153–154.

Macfie J & McMahon MJ (1980) The management of the open perineal wound using a foam elastomer: a prospective clinical trial. *British Journal of Surgery* 67: 85–89.

Foster ME & Williams P (1994) Wound healing — a surgical perspective. *Journal of Wound Care* 3(3): 135–138.

Morison PN, Corman ML & Collier JA (1976) Anterior resection for adenocarcinoma - Lahey clinical experience. *Diseases of the Colon and Rectum* 19: 219–224.

Malata CM, Williams NW & Shape DT (1995) Tissue expansion: an overview. *Journal of Wound Care* 4(1): 37–43.

Boore JRP, Champion R & Ferguson MC (1987) *Nursing the Physically Ill Adult. A Textbook of Medical-surgical Nursing*. Edinburgh: Churchill Livingstone.

References

Abelqvist J (1990) *Diabetic foot ulcers: the importance of clinical characteristics and prognostic factors for the outcome*. Department of Internal Medicine, University Hospital of Lund, Sweden.

Burkitt DP (1971) Epidemiology of cancer of the colon and rectum. *Cancer* 28: 3–13.

Connor H (1994) Prevention of diabetic foot problems. In: *The Foot in Diabetes*, 2nd edn. Chichester: John Wiley.

Fawcett JN *et al.* (1994) Diabetes. In: Alexander MF, Fawcett JN & Rincimon PJ (eds) *Nursing Practice, Hospital and Home. The Adult*. Edinburgh: Churchill Livingstone.

Foster A (1987) Examination of the diabetic foot — Part II. *Practical Diabetes* 4(4): 153–154.

Kelly H (1985) Loss and grief reactions as responses to surgery. *Journal of Advanced Nursing* 10: 517–525.

Liles L (1995) Stoma appliances: choices, prescription and problems. *Prescriber* Jan 5, 17–22.

McIntyre R (1994) Diabetes. In: Alexander MF, Fawcett JN & Rincimon PJ (eds) *Nursing Practice Hospital and Home. The Adult.* Edinburgh: Churchill Livingstone.

Miller R, Howie E & Murchie M (1994) The gastrointestinal system, liver and biliary tract. In: Alexander MF, Fawcett JN & Rincimon PJ (eds) *Nursing Practice Hospital and Home. The Adult.* Edinburgh: Churchill Livingstone.

Parker J (1994) The breast. In: Alexander MF, Fawcett JN & Rincimon PJ (eds) *Nursing Practice Hospital and Home. The Adult.* Edinburgh: Churchill Livingstone.

Tunbridge WH & Hare PP (1990) Diabetics and endocrinology. In: *Clinical Practice*, pp 56–57. London: Edward Arnold.

Walters DP, Gatling W, Mullee MA & Hill RD (1992) The distribution and severity of diabetic foot disease: a community study with comparison to a non-diabetic group. *Diabetic Medicine* 9: 354–358.

Williams DRR (1994) The size of the problem: epidemiological and economic aspects of feet problems in diabetes. In: Boulton AJM, Connor H & Cavanagh PR (eds) *The Foot in Diabetes*, 2nd edn. Chichester: John Wiley.

Willis J (1995) Stoma care, principles and product type. *Nursing Times* 91(2): 43–45.

Wound Healing Research Unit (1994) *Wound Management — Good Practice Guidance.* NHS Cymru Wales.

8 Wound Care in the Elderly Individual with a Pressure Sore

Key issues

This chapter deals with the particular problems associated with wound healing in the elderly individual.

Clinical Case Study

- The aetiology and management of a patient with a pressure sore cared for in a nursing home.

Nursing Model

- Roper's model is used as an example of its application to practice.

Practice points

As you read through this chapter concentrate on the following:

- Recognition of the predisposing factors that contribute to pressure sore development.
- Use of the appropriate risk assessment tool to assess patients at risk.
- Thorough assessment of the pressure sore to ensure appropriate wound management.
- Involvement of the multidisciplinary team in delivery of care.
- Use of appropriate equipment to meet individual needs.

Introduction

The management of elderly patients is one of the most challenging and ill-considered aspects of the life-cycle. Elderly patients with wounds often have a range of other problems which complicate their wound management.

Demographic changes are predicted to occur in the UK, with the numbers of elderly people rising rapidly, most growth being in the over-85 age group. Additionally, the number of people aged over 65 years, who currently make up 16% of the UK population, is expected to increase to 20.5% of the population by the year 2031 (Office of Health Economics 1992).

The prevalence of long-standing illnesses in people aged over 75 years is currently estimated at 70%, compared with only 35% in the total population. Such illnesses include circulatory diseases and arthritis. Diseases related to the elderly correlate with the development of pressure sores in hospitalized patients (David *et al.* 1993).

Problems Associated with Increasing Age

- Multiple disease processes
- Impaired mobility
- Slower metabolic processes
- Restricted (fixed) incomes
- Lack of medical resources due to finance problems
- Numbers of professional or lay persons to care for elderly

Pressure Sores

Pressure sores are a growing problem in an ageing population, and can easily arise in the situation described in Case Study 8.1.

Case Study 8.1
Pressure sores

Elsie Mason is an 83-year-old woman who, for the past 6 years, has been in residential care in a nursing home as her husband found it increasingly difficult to cope. Initially admitted for bouts of forgetfulness and inability to care for herself, her psychological condition deteriorated dramatically over the last 2 years and she has recently been diagnosed as having Alzheimer's disease. Whereas previously Elsie had been fairly mobile she has recently been difficult to mobilize and spends long periods in bed, often missing meals. She has also become incontinent of urine and faeces, failing to indicate to the staff when she wants to go to the toilet. She often is found wandering around at night and is becoming increasingly difficult to communicate with. Her husband is most distressed with her deterioration, especially as she often does not recognize him and tells people he is dead.

Three weeks ago, while Elsie was being bathed, a small red area was noticed on the left hip. Although this was thought insignificant at the time, within 4 days the whole of the hip had become blackened and lost the outer skin covering. Two weeks later a larger cavity some 12 cm by 10.2 cm and 2 cm deep appeared.

Epidemiology

Up to 20% of elderly patients being nursed in hospital have pressure sores (Norton *et al.* 1975). However, this figure rises to 30–50% in orthopaedic and care of the elderly wards (Hibbs 1982). In elderly patients an even higher incidence occurs in those patients admitted with fractured neck of femur, where the rate soars to 66% (Versluysen 1986).

One explanation for the increased incidence of pressure sores in the elderly is thought to be the increase in neurological and cardiovascular disorders, which are related to advanced age (Bliss 1990). Cardiovascular disorders adversely affect blood flow, especially to peripheral tissues, which is the main cause of pressure sores on the heel. Neurological disorders such as Alzheimer's disease and Parkinson's disease can impair mobility and sensation. In health the elderly person is highly unlikely to develop a pressure sore. It is when an elderly individual becomes ill they become extremely vulnerable to tissue damage. Such illness is likely to:

- lead to immobility or reduced mobility through spending time in bed, either at home or in hospital.
- mean admission to hospital where the patient may be nursed on a hard surface or spend time on X-ray, admission or theatre trolleys. In the elderly 15% of all sores are present on admission to hospital and 70% develop in the following 2 weeks, when such patients are most ill (Bliss 1990)
- reduced fluid intake and dehydration
- reduced food intake
- affect the cardiovascular system or neurological system
- produce incontinence

The above factors predispose the elderly, ill individual to developing pressure sores. Even when these factors are transient, tissue damage often has long-term consequences.

The implications for the health and well-being of the elderly patient who develops a pressure sore are serious: 50% of all elderly patients developing a pressure sore die within 4 months and this rises to 90% when patients develop necrotic pressure sores on the trunk (Bliss 1990). With this in mind it is sobering to note that it has been estimated that 95% of pressure sores are preventable (Waterlow 1988).

The personal cost to the individual is high in terms of morbidity and mortality, but pressure sores are also a drain on financial resources. The cost of managing pressure sores is vast and continues to rise. In the UK the estimated annual cost was around £60 million in 1973, £150 million in 1982 (Scales *et al.* 1982) and £300 million in 1988 (Waterlow 1988). The UK, however, is not an isolated case. In the USA the cost of treating a patient in hospital with a pressure sore ranges from $2000 to $30 000 (Eaglestein 1990). Currently around a million patients are treated for pressure sores in the USA annually, compared with 30 000 in the UK (Duthie 1990). By the year 2030 it is projected that 60 million Americans (20%) will be over the age of 65 years. In the UK, by the year 2025, about 25% of the population will be over 65 years (Scales 1990). The projected elderly population for the UK can be seen in Figure 8.1.

Figure 8.1   *Projections of the elderly population. From OHE Compendium of Health Statistics (1992). Note projections based on 1989 mid year estimates. Source: Annual Abstract of Statistics.*

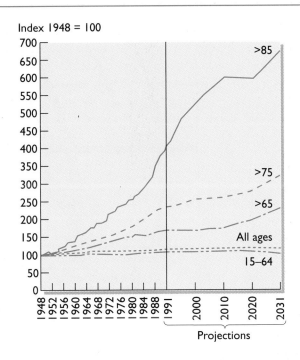

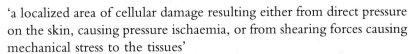

Aetiology

Although many nurses feel sure that they know exactly what constitutes a pressure sore, it can be difficult to define the term. Chapman and Chapman (1986) used the following definition:

> 'a localized area of cellular damage resulting either from direct pressure on the skin, causing pressure ischaemia, or from shearing forces causing mechanical stress to the tissues'

A clinical practice guide in the USA (Banks 1992) uses a more simplified definition:

> 'a pressure ulcer is any lesion caused by unrelieved pressure resulting in damage of underlying tissue'

Banks (1992) brought together several definitions:

> 'a pressure sore is an area of localized damage to the skin and may involve underlying structures. Tissue damage can be restricted to superficial epidermal loss or extend to involve muscle and bone'

Normal skin

A brief overview of the structure and functions of normal, healthy, undamaged skin follows to help understand the pathogenesis and pathophysiology of pressure sore development.

The skin is made up of two layers, the epidermis and the dermis (Figure 8.2). The outer epidermal layer is a barrier, preventing the evaporation of

Figure 8.2 *Structure of the skin.*

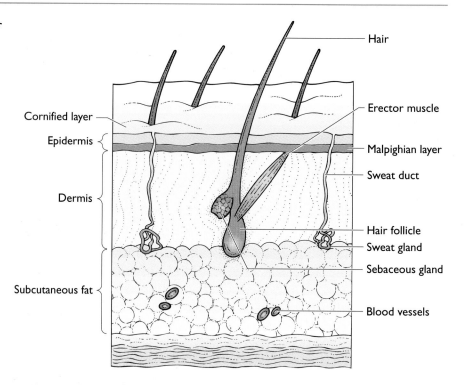

Cornified layer

Epidermis

Dermis

Subcutaneous fat

Hair

Erector muscle

Malpighian layer

Sweat duct

Hair follicle

Sweat gland

Sebaceous gland

Blood vessels

water from the body and conversely preventing absorption of water from the outside environment. The dermal layer also forms a physical barrier preventing the access of bacteria.

The epidermis consists of dead keratinized cells; these cells are continually being shed from the body and are continually replaced from the base of the epidermis. The deeper dermal layer contains blood capillaries, sweat glands, hair follicles and nerve endings. The main functions of the dermis are sensory perception, the control of body temperature and the spread of pressure. This dermal layer varies in thickness, and the skin's ability to spread pressure varies with the thickness.

In healthy individuals, the blood supply to the skin delivers vital oxygen and nutrients and normal sensation is experienced. Pressure sores result when healthy tissues become devitalized so causing localized tissue death. Pressure sores are known to develop in several ways:

i)   When direct, unrelieved pressure occurs over bony areas. Pressure can be defined as the force exerted perpendicularly over a given area, divided by that area. Duration of pressure is very important. Tissue damage can occur when high pressure is exerted over an area for a short period, or (more often) when lower pressures occur over a prolonged period. The areas covering the bony prominences of the human skeleton are susceptible to such damage owing to there being little tissue to spread the pressure.

ii)   When friction occurs between the patient's tissues and the hard surface of a bed or chair (Figure 8.3). Typically this can happen when a patient is mishandled and dragged up a bed when being repositioned.

iii) When shear force occurs. Shear force is often experienced in combina-

Figure 8.3 *Common sites for pressure sore development: (a) sitting in bed, (b) lying in bed, (c) sitting in a chair.*

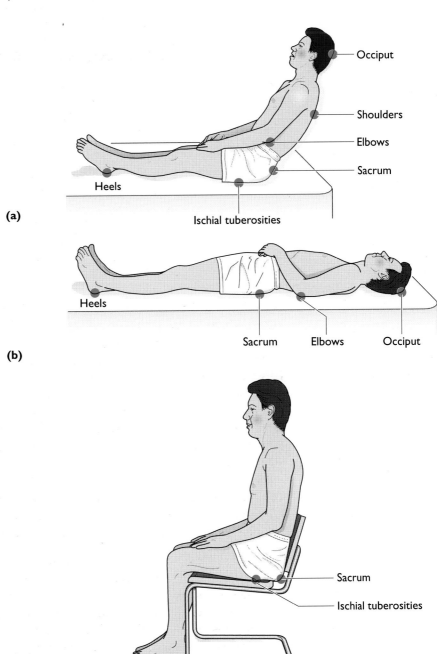

Figure 8.4   *Sites of pressure sores. (Percentages are from Dealey, 1991.)*

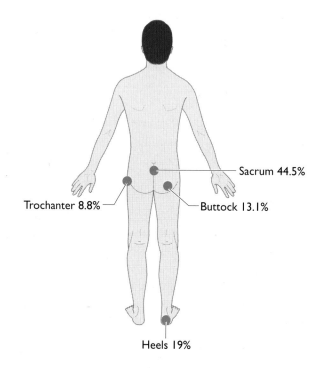

Sacrum 44.5%

Trochanter 8.8%

Buttock 13.1%

Heels 19%

tion with friction and direct pressure, and happens when tissues are pulled and distorted, disrupting the blood supply to that area. As with pressure, the duration of the shearing is important. Although rigorous shearing can cause tissue necrosis, repeated shearing at a lower level also causes severe tissue damage.

A number of research projects have shown the usual location and distribution of pressure sores. Although some variation exists, the sacrum, buttocks and trochanters are particularly susceptible to pressure sore development, which often results from sitting in a chair rather than from being nursed in bed (Figure 8.4).

Classification of Pressure Sores

Classification or grading of pressure sores is based on the degree of tissue damage observed. Several classifications are available; a small selection of the most commonly used systems are described here.

Hibbs classification

The following classification was proposed by Hibbs (1988).

- Stage I — blanching hyperaemia. Reactive hyperaemia causes a distinct erythema after pressure is released. Light finger pressure will cause blanching of this erythema, indicating that the microcirculation is intact.

- Stage II — non-blanching hyperaemia. Erythema remains after release of pressure. A degree of microcirculatory disruption and inflammation, oedema and thickening occurs. Superficial swelling, induration, blistering and epidermal ulceration will be present.

- Stage III — ulceration progresses through to the subcutaneous tissue. Ulcer edges are distinct, but surrounded by erythema and induration. At this stage damage is still reversible (Figure 8.5).

- Stage IV — lesion extends to subcutaneous fat. Small vessel thrombosis and infection compound fat necrosis. There is a distinct ulcer margin, but lateral extension of necrosis continues under the skin. Deep fascia temporarily impedes downward progress.

- Stage V — infective necrosis. Necrosis penetrates the deep fascia and muscle induration proceeds rapidly. Joints and body cavities can become involved. Multiple sores may communicate.

- Closed pressure sores — there is deep, extensive damage to tissues, but the surface presents as a small ulcer.

NPUAP classification

The National Pressure Ulcer Advisory Panel (NPUAP 1989) recommended a classification into four stages.

- Stage I — non-blanchable erythema of intact skin: the heralding lesion of skin ulceration.

- Stage II — partial-thickness skin loss involving epidermis and possibly also the dermis. The ulcer is superficial and presents clinically as an abrasion, blister or shallow crater (Figure 8.6).

- Stage III — full-thickness skin loss involving damage or necrosis of subcutaneous tissue that may extend down to, but not through, under-lying fascia. The ulcer presents clinically as a deep crater with or without undermining of adjacent tissue (Figure 8.7).

- Stage IV — full-thickness skin loss with extensive destruction, tissue necrosis or damage to muscle, bone or supporting structures (for example, tendon or joint capsule). Undermining and sinus tracts may also be associated with stage IV pressure ulcers (Figure 8.8).

UK consensus committee classification

In the UK a consensus committee has been formed to review existing classifications, identify practical problems encountered with their use and produce a national classification to achieve a common standard for documentation (Reid and Morison 1994). This classification system grades pressure sores into four stages. In addition it uses four digits: the first two digits describe the level and nature of tissue involvement, the third digit

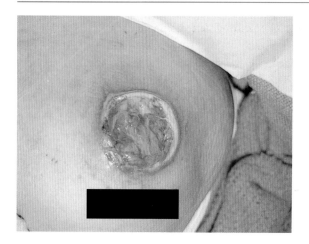

Figure 8.5   *Stage III pressure sore with a soft, sloughy wound bed.*

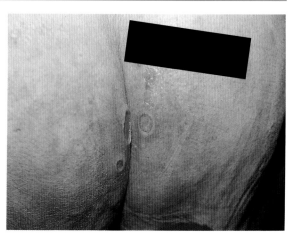

Figure 8.6   *Stage II pressure sore.*

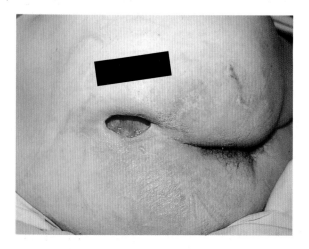

Figure 8.7   *Stage III pressure sore.*

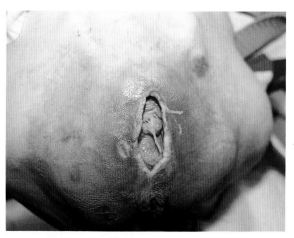

Figure 8.8   *Stage IV pressure sore.*

relates to the nature of the wound bed and the fourth allows for coding of infective complications. It is hoped that this system, if used in the UK, will provide a common language for describing pressure sores.

Prevention of Pressure Sores

Most pressure sores are preventable (Waterlow 1988). Working on the principle that prevention is better than cure, prevention of pressure sores is discussed before treatment and management.

Assessment of risk

Identification of those elderly individuals susceptible to developing pressure sores is the first and most important step in preventing tissue breakdown.

Table 8.1   *What makes older people susceptible to tissue damage?*

The onset of an intercurrent illness or trauma

Immobility, e.g. through illness or orthopaedic surgery

Sensory impairment, e.g. diabetes, comatosis, neurological disease

Systemic disease, e.g. carcinoma, cardiovascular disease, anaemia

Incontinence

Dehydration

Poor nutrition, malnutrition

Patients either below or above average body weight

Unrelieved pressure, friction, shearing

Clearly, not all elderly people have pressure sores: so what exactly increases the risk? Important factors are listed in Table 8.1.

Many pressure sore risk assessment tools have been devised. Some of these are specifically aimed for use with elderly patients, the first — and probably the simplest — being the Norton scale (Norton *et al.* 1975) shown in Table 8.2.

Later and more comprehensive scales take into account more factors. One example is the Waterlow scoring system. Shown in Table 8.3 (Waterlow 1988). This scoring system is available on a washable, plastic card which allows for reuse and easy reassessment.

In the USA in 1988 the Braden scale, based on the Norton scale, was introduced; it is probably the most popular scoring system used in the USA.

Nutritional issues in the elderly

In the healthy, elderly individual all tissue is constantly being remodelled or repaired. In the well-nourished individual there is ready availability of proteins, carbohydrates and fats, together with the necessary vitamins and minerals needed for cell metabolism. Poor nutrition interferes with normal metabolic processes so predisposing the elderly to pressure sore formation. When this leads also to weight loss there is less padding over the bony prominences, so increasing the risk of pressure sore development. The nutritional needs of the young and old are identical, apart from energy

Table 8.2 *The Norton scale for calculating pressure sore risk. A total score of 14 or below indicates that the patient is at risk*

Physical condition	Mental state	Activity	Mobility	Incontinence
4 Good	4 Alert	4 Ambulant	4 Full	4 None
3 Fair	3 Apathetic	3 Walks with help	3 Slightly limited	3 Occasional
2 Poor	2 Confused	2 Chairbound	2 Very limited	2 Usually urinary
1 Very bad	1 Stuporous	1 Bedfast	1 Immobile	1 Double

Table 8.3   *Waterlow pressure sore prevention/treatment policy*

BUILD/WEIGHT FOR HEIGHT	★	SKIN TYPE VISUAL RISK AREAS	★	SEX AGE	★	SPECIAL RISKS	★
Average	0	Healthy	0	MALE	1	**TISSUE MALNUTRITION**	★
Above average	1	Tissue paper	1	FEMALE	2		
Obese	2	Dry	1	14–49	1	e.g. Terminal cachexia	8
Below average	3	Oedematous	1	50–64	2	Cardiac failure	5
		Clammy (temp ↑)	1	65–74	3	Peripheral vascular	
CONTINENCE	★	Discoloured	2	75–80	4	disease	5
		Broken/spot	3	81+	5	Anaemia	2
Complete/						Smoking	1
Catheterized	0	**MOBILITY**	★	**APPETITE**	★	**NEUROLOGICAL DEFICIT**	★
Occasion incontinent	1						
Cath/incontinent		Fully mobile	0	Average	0	eg: Diabetes, M.S. CVA,	
of faeces	2	Restless/fidgety	1	Poor	1	Motor/sensory	4–6
Doubly incontinent	3	Apathetic	2	N.g. tube/		Paraplegia	
		Restricted	3	Fluids only	2		
		Inert/traction	4	Nbm/anorexic	3	**MAJOR SURGERY/TRAUMA**	★
		Chairbound	5				
						Orthopaedic –	
						Below waist, spinal	5
						On table > 2 hours	5

SCORE	10+ AT RISK	15+ HIGH RISK	20+ VERY HIGH RISK

MEDICATION	★
Cytotoxic drugs	4
High dose steroids	
Anti-inflammatory drugs	

RING SCORES IN TABLE, ADD TOTAL. SEVERAL SCORES PER CATEGORY CAN BE USED
N.g. nasogastric

© J Waterlow 1991 Revised May 1995

requirements. The elderly are generally less active and so require less energy (Table 8.4) and also have a reduced basal metabolic rate (Barker 1991).

The elderly population has been identified as a high-risk group for becoming malnourished (McLaren 1992). Many factors, including lack of motivation, low income and increasing frailty, account for poor-quality food intake. Malnutrition can also be difficult to detect and measure. It is possible that many elderly individuals have some degree of subclinical malnutrition.

Apart from the need for appropriate intakes of protein, carbohydrate and fat, some vitamins and minerals are specifically linked with wound healing. It has been suggested that supplements of certain elements increase the rate of tissue repair but there is, as yet, no sound evidence that high doses of any one

Table 8.4   *Changes in energy requirements for men and women*

Age (years)	Men (Kcal)	(kJ)	Women (Kcal)	(kJ)
18	3 000	12 600	2 200	9 240
75+	2 100	8 820	1 900	7 980

Table 8.5 *Simple changes to improve the diet of the elderly*

1. Have a glass of fruit juice every day
2. Have a fortified wholegrain cereal (e.g. Weetabix) with milk for breakfast
3. Try to eat meat or fish once every day
4. Have a milk drink at bedtime
5. Eat at least one serving of vegetables every day

From Barker (1991).

nutrient will do this (Dickenson 1993). Ascorbic acid (vitamin C) and zinc are two such substances. Vitamin C and zinc deficiency can prevent or delay healing. The UK recommended daily intake for vitamin C is 40 mg and for zinc is 9.5 mg in men and 7 mg in women (Department of Health 1991). The blood values of vitamin C and zinc are so difficult to measure that it has been suggested (Dickenson 1993) that where deficiencies are suspected in the elderly (through dietary, social history and physical condition) treatment is probably beneficial. For patients with pressure sores, 1000 mg of vitamin C can be given. As the renal threshold for vitamin C is low this should be given in four 250 mg doses throughout the day (Dickenson 1993). Zinc also is given three divided doses of 220 mg. Malnutrition is a real problem for the elderly. In a prevalence survey carried out by Pinchcofsky-Devin and Kaminski (1986), the overall incidence of malnutrition in the elderly was 59%. This survey also categorized the degree of malnutrition as mild, moderate or severe, and found that the elderly patients with pressure sores were all in the severely malnourished group.

When caring for the elderly it may be pertinent to think about the possibility of poor nutrition or malnutrition carefully. With a few simple changes it is possible to improve the diet of an elderly individual (Table 8.5).

Practice points

- Perhaps you have an elderly relative. Find out what their average intake of food is. Look at the whole week. Is the diet balanced and is adequate energy being consumed?
- The next time you are working in this clinical area, select one patient and keep an accurate record of how much and what type of foods the patient is eating.

Equipment for the relief of pressure

A vast array of equipment is available for the relief of pressure, at a wide range of costs. It is therefore understandable that much confusion surrounds this issue. Dealey (1992) classified patients into low, medium and high-risk categories and described a range of pressure relieving devices for these groups:

- Low-risk patients:
    sheepskins
    hollow-core fibre pads
    bead overlays
    foam overlays
    gel pads
- Medium-risk patients:
    foam overlays
    foam replacement mattresses
    combination foam/water mattresses
    combination foam/gel mattresses
    alternating air pads
    water beds
    double-layer alternating air pads
- High-risk patients:
    double-layer alternating air pads
    air-flotation pads
    dynamic air-flotation mattresses
    air-wave mattresses
    air-fluidized bed

Considering most pressure sores could be prevented, very few resources are utilized to encourage and motivate nurses, carers and elderly individuals towards prevention.

Assessment of the Elderly Patient with a Pressure Sore

An elderly individual who has developed a pressure sore requires a thorough assessment and rapid nursing intervention. Owing to the nature of the wound it is inappropriate to deliver a local wound treatment without considering both the physical condition of the elderly individual and the environment in which care is provided. There is a sense of urgency, as the main aim is to prevent further tissue damage while promoting healing. This assessment process precedes the development of a management plan and delivery of care.

Questions to Ask

Nutritional status

Albumin
a water-soluble protein. Serum albumin is the chief protein of blood plasma.

- Has the patient been receiving adequate nutrition in the past, and is the patient currently receiving adequate nutrition? (see above)
- Has the patient's serum **albumin** level been determined? If so, does the level lie within the normal range?
- Does the nutrition of this patient need to be improved?
- Should the dietician be consulted for advice?

Continence

- Is the patient continent of urine and faeces?
- If yes — what can be done to maintain continence?
- If no — how can continence be promoted?
- Should catheterization be considered?
- What types of incontinence aids are available?

Mobility

- What range of mobility does this patient have — full, restricted, limited or none?
- Could mobility be improved with an aid, e.g. Zimmer frame, walking stick, tripod?
- Would physiotherapy help improve mobility?
- What motivation is there to move?

Pressure relief

- What pressure-relieving devices are currently being used to reduce pressure, e.g. foam overlay mattress, chair cushion?
- Is this appropriate for the needs of this patient?
- What is the optimum system for this patient and is it available?
- Does the patient have other areas that are showing signs of pressure?

Wound Assessment

A careful examination of the pressure sore should be undertaken to determine:

- Wound site
- The extent of tissue damage
- Wound measurement
- The health of the wound bed

Wound site

A chart showing a simple outline of the body can be used to record the site of a pressure sore. If more than one sore is present, these can be numbered on the chart for more accurate documentation.

The extent of tissue damage

Whatever classification system is used (see above), the grade of pressure sore should be assessed and documented directly onto the body chart and/or separately in the nursing notes.

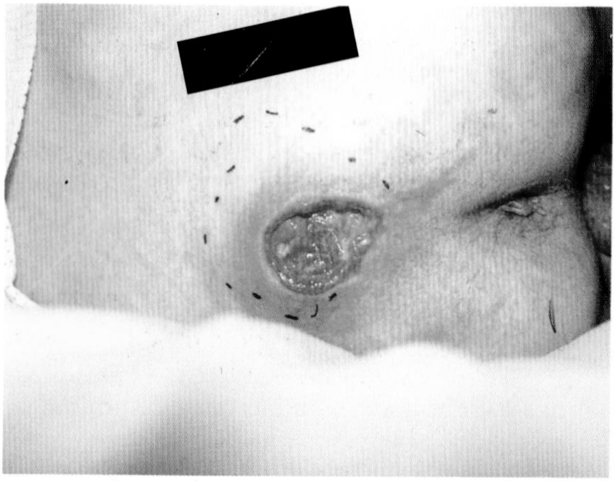

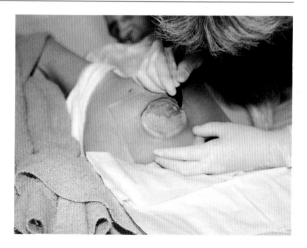

Figure 8.9 *Mapping on the skin of a patient with sacral pressure sore which shows the undermined area of tissue damage.*

Figure 8.10 *Wound measurement: taking a tracing of a pressure sore.*

Wound measurement

Measurement of pressure sores can be difficult owing to the problems associated with poor wound shape. Tissue damage can spread laterally, undermining the skin (Figure 8.9). The problems associated with undermining include:

- Poor exudate drainage predisposing to wound infection and odour
- The possibility of further, devitalized tissue being present which cannot be seen
- Difficulties in dressing management

An accurate as possible estimation of wound size will help in monitoring the progress or deterioration of the pressure sore. Where no undermining or depth occurs, a tracing can be taken (Figure 8.10). Where undermining occurs, the wound opening can be traced, together with the undermined area denoted with a broken line using forceps to determine the extent of the damage.

Health of the wound bed

The appearance of the wound bed is essential in determining the health of the tissues. A range of tissues may be encountered (see Chapter 1):

i)   Healthy pink or yellow granulation tissue.
ii)   Devitalized tissue, indicating that full wound debridement is not complete.
iii)   Infected tissue. The clinical signs of wound infection are described in Chapter 1. Pressure sores are likely to become infected owing to the presence of damaged tissue.
iv)   Dry wound bed: when a pressure sore is exposed to the air for long

periods the surface dries out; wound healing can be impaired in the absence of a moist environment.

v) Excessively exuding wounds: when large amounts of wound exudate are produced, for example by very extensive pressure sores, the skin surrounding the sore is susceptible to further tissue damage from becoming macerated.

Meticulous assessment and documentation form the first part of caring for an elderly patient with a pressure sore. Further tissue damage should have been eliminated by this stage and management can proceed.

Wound Management

Having addressed the issues of nutrition, continence, mobility and risk of further tissue damage, the specific management of the pressure sore can begin. Although many of the general principles for managing a cavity wound should be taken into account, some additional points require special reference.

- Management of a necrotic pressure sore (Figure 8.11). Although this tissue appears to indicate superficial damage, the reverse is often true. Figure 8.12 shows what is happening beneath the surface. Pressure against the bone has caused extensive tissue damage, which has spread laterally. The necrotic area is relatively small, and many nurses are surprised that once treatment is initiated the sore rapidly extends, revealing an extensive wound (Figure 8.13). Hydrogel and hydrocolloid materials are useful dressings to effect wound debridement in this type of pressure sore. The moistness of these products rehydrates the necrotic area, so facilitating autolysis of the devitalized from the healthy tissue. Over a period of 7–14 days, as the devitalized tissue is removed, the wound may get alarmingly bigger. What is actually happening is that the devitalized tissue which was already damaged has been removed.

- Management of undermining (Figure 8.12c). Once the extent of the sore has been determined and documented, a material to pack the sore under the skin edges is needed. Hard materials such as gauze packing should be avoided as these materials cause further pressure. Dressing materials such as alginate packing, hydrogel, hydrocolloid pastes and hydrocellular foam cavity dressings fill the undermining area while creating an environment conducive to healing.

A flow chart outlining some of the basic steps to take when managing the older individual with, or at risk of developing, a pressure sore is shown in Figure 8.14.

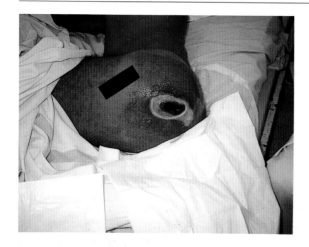

Figure 8.11   *Wound bed with necrotic tissue.*

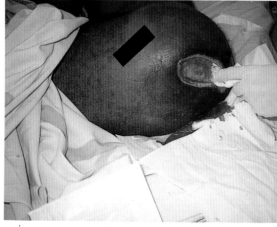

Figure 8.13   *The necrotic area is removed revealing the full extent of tissue damage.*

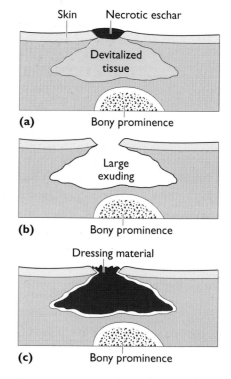

Figure 8.12   *Management of a necrotic pressure sore: (a) extent of the damage; (b) necrotic area removed, revealing full extent of the tissue damage; (c) dressing material fills the undermining cavity, but is not packed too tightly.*

Figure 8.14   *Flow chart outlining the management of an older individual with (or at risk of developing) a pressure sore.*

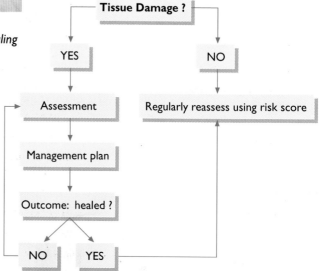

Nursing model for Elsie

It is obvious from Elsie's case study that her interaction with her carers has decreased and that she is often unable to participate actively in her care. When assessing Elsie's problems, the goals should relate to helping her cope with her dependencies in an attempt to achieve some independence.

A number of models could be used for Elsie, but probably one of the systems models such as that of Roper *et al.* (1980), which stresses the physical side of nursing would be best suited to a patient like Elsie. Although each part is studied separately, the interaction between these parts is most important.

As always, the nurse must set priorities of care when using the twelve assessment areas. Although the wound may seem the most important area, the potential for healing will be impaired if Elsie's nutritional status is ignored. Remember, too, that Elsie is being cared for in a nursing home, where levels of trained staff may be low. Care should be straightforward and manageable for all involved.

The assessment of Elsie's activities of living is given in Table 8.6, and the care plan in Table 8.7.

Table 8.6   *Assessment of Elsie's usual routine (Case Study 8.1)*

Activity of living	Problem statement
Maintaining a safe environment	Often wanders around at night
Communicating	Slightly deaf, wears glasses Does not communicate clearly, often talks to herself, does not recognize people
Breathing	Breathes easily, no chest problems Blood pressure within normal limits
Eating and drinking	Malnourished Needs to be reminded and encouraged to eat and drink Lacks interest in food — 'plays' with it
Eliminating	Incontinent of urine during day and night Occasionally incontinent of faeces at night
Personal cleansing and dressing	Will sometimes wash herself Often dresses without regard to items Skin often excoriated with urine
Controlling body temperature	Normal temperature
Mobilizing	Spends long periods of time in bed Has pressure sore on right hip
Working and playing	Sometimes joins in with home's activities but often sits by herself
Expressing sexuality	Does not always recognize husband, thinks he is dead on occasions
Sleeping	Often awake during the night, sleeps during the day
Dying	Expresses wish to die on occasions

Table 8.7　Care plan based on problems identified in Table 8.6

Activity of living	Problem	Goal	Intervention
Mobilizing	Pressure sore cavity 6 cm × 2 cm containing necrotic tissue (A)	Promote healing with removal of necrotic tissue	Debride wound with combined use of hydrogel and surgical debridement
	Infection in cavity (P)	Eliminate infection	1. Take wound swab 2. Doctor to prescribe appropriate antibiotics 3. Apply principles of asepsis; avoid cross-contamination
	Lacks motivation to mobilize (A)	Prevent shear forces and direct pressure	Involve Elsie in the home's activities. Encourage mixing with other residents
	Further skin breakdown (P)	1. Keep skin clean 2. Promote wound healing 3. Eliminate extrinsic factors	1. Assess with Risk Assessment Tool 2. Instal appropriate pressure-relieving equipment 3. Change position and mobilize 2-hourly during day, change position 4-hourly at nights. Daily shower or bath. Ensure all staff familiar with regimen
Eating and drinking	Malnourished (A) Further protein breakdown (P)	1. Counteract effects of catabolism 2. Promote wound healing	1. Refer to community dietician for assessment 2. Give 3000–4000 Kcal (1260–1680 kJ) with high-protein supplement 3. Staff to monitor mealtimes
Eliminating	Incontinent of urine and faeces (A) Skin maceration increasing risk of friction (P)	1. Restore continence 2. Prevent further skin breakdown	1. Staff to toilet Elsie every 2 hours 2. Rule out urinary tract infection or faecal retention 3. Avoid drinks before bedtime, toilet before bedtime 4. Wash skin thoroughly if contaminated 5. Avoid use of incontinence sheets or pads
Communicating	Difficulty in communicating needs	Maintain level of reality orientation	1. Speak clearly and always talk in the present 2. Avoid use of reminiscence 3. Inform Elsie of all nursing actions, involving her husband in care where possible 4. Ensure husband understands the nature of the disease process
Sleeping	Disturbed sleep pattern (A)	Restore normal pattern of 6 hours per night	1. Keep Elsie active in the daytime 2. Do not allow her to sleep during the day 3. Establish a bedtime routine
Expressing sexuality	Husband separated from wife — feels guilty at leaving her in a nursing home	Restore role for husband	Give husband tasks to aid his wife's recovery, e.g. feeding at mealtimes, and toileting during the day

(A), actual problem; (P), potential problem.

Practice points

- It is important to note that, although the care for Elsie was comprehensive, she is at constant risk of developing further sores, as are many of the other residents in the home.
- Education is an important factor for the staff of the home, and community nursing input should aim to provide a programme of support and advice to the matron and staff.

Summary

There is much to think about in order that patients are managed with the optimum level of care. Management requires the skill and expertise of many health team members, whether the patient is in hospital or the community. It is important that you become a team member and learn when to use the other team members' expertise, e.g.

- Dietician — ensures type and level of protein and carbohydrates appropriate to patient's needs
- Occupational therapist — supplies pressure-relieving equipment
- Physiotherapist — ensures muscle wasting and contractures are kept to a minimum
- Tissue viability nurse — available for specialist advice, and may be responsible for protocol development
- Plastic surgeon — required for healing of pressure sores
- Physician, surgeon — controls intrinsic factors such as diabetes, urinary incontinence
- Generalist nurse — coordinates plan of care; educates patient and relatives

A planned programme of care will include all these people. Recognition of predisposing factors and early signs of pressure sore development outlined in this chapter will contribute to the lowering of the incidence and prevalence of pressure sores.

Could *you* recognize them?

Further Reading

Bader DL (1990) *Pressure Sores. Clinical Practice and Scientific Approach.* London: Macmillan.

Versluysen M (1986) How elderly patients with femoral neck fractures develop pressure sores in hospital. *British Medical Journal* 292: 1311–1313.

Norton D, McLaron R & Exton-Smith AV (1975) *An Investigation of Geriatric Nursing Problems in Hospital.* Edinburgh: Churchill Livingstone.

Barton A & Barton M (1978) *The Management and Prevention of Pressure Sores.* London: Faber & Faber.

Torrance C (1983) *Pressure Sores: Aetiology, Treatment and Prevention.* London: Croom Helm.

Krasner D, ed. (1990) *Chronic Wound Care: A Clinical Source Book for Healthcare Professionals.* King of Prussia, Pa: Health Management.

References

Banks V (1992) Pressure sores: a community problem. *Journal of Wound Care.* 1(2): 42–44.

Barker HM (1991) Nutrition and the elderly. *Beck's Nutrition and Dietetics for Nurses.* Edinburgh: Churchill Livingstone.

Bliss M (1990) Geriatric medicine. In: Bader DL (ed.) *Pressure Sores. Clinical Practice and Scientific Approach.* London: Macmillan.

Chapman EJ & Chapman R (1986) Treatment of pressure sores: the state of the art. In: Tierney AJ (ed.) *Clinical Nursing Practice,* Recent Advances in Nursing Series, Edinburgh: Churchill Livingstone.

David G, Chapman RG, Chapman EZ *et al.* (1983) *An investigation of the current methods used in nursing for the care of patients with established pressure sores.* Harrow: Nursing Practice Unit.

Dealey C (1991) The size of the pressure sore problem in a teaching hospital. *Journal of Advanced Nursing.* 16: 633–670.

Dealey C (1992) How are you supporting your patients? A review of pressure relieving equipment. In: Horne EM *et al.* (eds) *Staff Nurses' Survival Guide,* 2nd edn. London: Wolfe.

Department of Health (1991) Dietary reference values for food, energy and nutrients for the United Kingdom. *Report of Health and Social Subjects 41.* London: HMSO.

Dickenson JWT (1993) Ascorbic acid, zinc and wound healing. *Journal of Wound Care* 2(6): 350–353.

Duthie R (1990) Foreword. In: Bader DL (ed.) *Pressure Sores: Clinical Practice and Scientific Approach.* London: Macmillan.

Eaglestein W (1990) *New Directions in Wound Healing.* Convatec: New Jersey.

Hibbs P (1982) Pressure sores: a system of prevention. *Nursing Mirror* 155(5): 25–29.

Hibbs P (1988) *Pressure Area Care for the City and Hackney Health Authority.* City and Hackney Health Authority.

McLaren SMG (1992) Nutrition and wound healing. *Journal of Wound Care* 1(3): 45–55.

National Pressure Ulcer Advisory Panel (1989) Pressure ulcers prevalence, cost and risk assessment. Consensus Development Conference statement. *Decubitus* 2: 24–35.

Norton D, McLaren R & Exton-Smith AN (1975) *An Investigation of Geriatric Nursing Problems in Hospital.* Edinburgh: Churchill Livingstone.

Office of Health Economics (1992) *Compendium of Health Care Statistics.* London: OHE.

Pinchcofsky-Devin GD & Kaminski MV (1986) Correlation of pressure sores and nutritional status. *Journal of the American Geriatric Society* 34: 435–440.

Reid J & Morison M (1994) Towards a consensus classification of pressure sores. *Journal of Wound Care* 3(3): 151–160.

Roper N, Logan W & Tierney A (1980) *The Elements of Nursing.* Edinburgh: Churchill Livingstone.

Scales JT (1990) Pathogenesis of pressure sores. In: Bader DL (ed.) *Pressure Sores: Clinical Practice and Scientific Approach.* London: Macmillan.

Scales JT, Lowthian PJ & Poole AG (1982) 'Vaperm' patient support system: a new general purpose hospital mattress. *Lancet* 2: 1150–1152.

Versluysen M (1986) How elderly patients with femoral neck fractures develop pressure sores in hospital. *British Medical Journal* 292: 1311–1313.

Waterlow J (1988) Prevention is cheaper than cure. *Nursing Times* 84(25): 69–70.

Wound Care in the Elderly Individual with Leg Ulceration and Malignancy

Key issues

This chapter looks at wounds other than pressure sores that are common in the elderly population.

Clinical Case Studies

Aetiology and management of:

- An independent woman suffering with venous ulceration
- The onset of arterial ulceration in an elderly man
- Advanced stages of breast disease in a lady with a fungating breast tumour

Practice points

As you read through this chapter, concentrate on the following:

- the importance of the nurse–patient relationship in helping patients understand the nature of their wounds
- the importance of correct assessment when dealing with patients with leg ulceration
- palliative management of a wound when healing is not the outcome
- the importance of understanding the basic principles of wound management

Introduction

The general problems of wound management in the elderly patient were discussed in the introduction to Chapter 8. This chapter concentrates on the problems of leg ulceration and malignancy.

Leg Ulceration

It has been estimated that in 1992 around 400 000 patients in the UK had experienced leg ulceration, 100 000 of whom currently required treatment (Fletcher 1992). Leg ulceration affects about 0.15% of the population in the

Table 9.1   *Increasing prevalence of leg ulcers in women with advancing age*

Age (years)	Male–female ratio
under 65	1:1
65–74	1:2.6
75–84	1:4.8
85+	1:10.3

From Callam *et al* (1987).

UK (Callam *et al.* 1985), and the prevalence increases with age, from 10 per 1000 within the adult population to 36 per 1000 in the over-65 age group — particularly in women (Table 9.1).

The estimated costs of treating leg ulcer patients ranges from £150 million to £600 million per annum in the UK (Wilson 1989). A high proportion of these costs are spent on dressings and district nurse time, with district nurses spending 10–50% of their time managing leg ulcer patients (Moffatt and Morison 1994). Only 1% of leg ulcer patients are managed in hospital (Callam *et al.* 1985). The implications of this are that patients with leg ulceration are treated in the community, with district nurses providing day-to-day care for these patients and also acting as a facilitator for other services.

The aetiology of leg ulcers is shown in Figure 9.1. One per cent of these ulcers may be malignant (Figure 9.2).

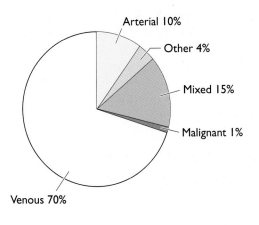

Arterial 10%
Other 4%
Mixed 15%
Malignant 1%
Venous 70%

Figure 9.1   *Aetiology of leg ulcers.*

Figure 9.2   *A malignant ulcer.*

Venous Ulcers

In the elderly population, venous disease is the major cause of leg ulceration. A case of venous ulceration is described in Case Study 9.1.

Case Study 9.1
Venous ulcers

Joan Knight, an independent 73-year-old retired headteacher, is an active member of the village community in which she has lived and taught all her life. Although now widowed and living alone, she has much social contact. While helping to serve tea at the local summer fête she scraped her leg on the tea trolley. The laceration bled profusely, but having enlisted the aid of a friend to stop the bleeding, Joan thought no more about it. She treated the wound herself with an old remedy of cold tea soaks and a bandage, but was dismayed to find that 6 weeks later the wound had developed into a deep crater which was producing lots of exudate and smelt rather unpleasant.

She reluctantly went to her general practitioner who seemed to be more interested in asking her about when she had had her children than the wound itself. Joan recalled that after the birth of both children she had a condition called 'white leg'.

The doctor sent her to the district nurse's room, where blood was taken, the wound measured and the ankle brachial pressure index in the affected leg was recorded.

Aetiology

In health the venous system of the lower leg pumps blood back towards the heart. As this action takes place against gravity in the human this is difficult to achieve.

There are three categories of vein within the legs: deep, superficial and communicating (perforator) veins. The superficial long and short saphenous veins (draining the skin) pump blood under low pressure into the deep venous system through the perforators (Figure 9.3). The deep veins are surrounded by muscles (the calf muscle pump) which contract and relax during walking to pump blood up the leg. Healthy venous return is achieved not only by walking (so using the calf muscle pump) but also by having full ankle movement — when the ankle moves the Achilles tendon contracts and releases, to assist the calf muscle pump.

Damage to the venous system can occur at any time of life. Deep vein thrombosis and varicose veins damage the perforators, making them incompetent (Figure 9.4). Immobility of, and arthritic changes to, the ankle joint impair ankle movement and so further impede venous return.

Back flow of blood results in venous hypertension, which leads to oedema of the lower leg and pigmentation of the 'gaiter' area. This pigmentation (lipodermatosclerosis) is the result of haemoglobin being released from red blood cells which have leaked out of the distended blood capillaries. A fibrin cuff forms around these capillaries and has the effect of interfering with oxygen diffusion into the tissues. Any subsequent knock or minor injury to this area of the lower leg can rapidly lead to ulceration. Ulceration most commonly found occurs around the gaiter area (Figure 9.5) where usually

Figure 9.3 *The normal venous system of the leg.*

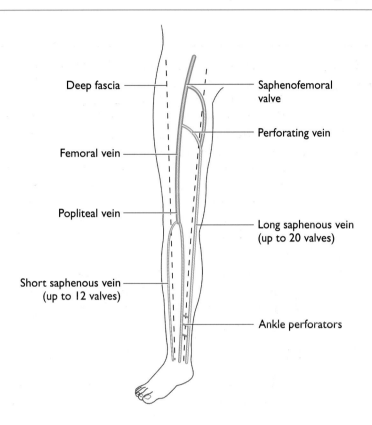

Deep fascia

Saphenofemoral valve

Perforating vein

Femoral vein

Popliteal vein

Long saphenous vein (up to 20 valves)

Short saphenous vein (up to 12 valves)

Ankle perforators

Figure 9.4 *A damaged venous system: an incompetent valve in a perforating vein allows backflow of blood from the deep to the superficial venous system.*

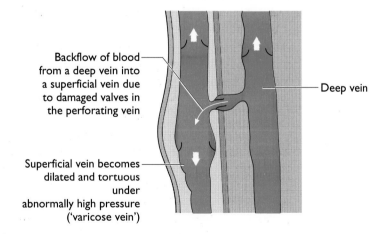

Backflow of blood from a deep vein into a superficial vein due to damaged valves in the perforating vein

Deep vein

Superficial vein becomes dilated and tortuous under abnormally high pressure ('varicose vein')

the ulcers are shallow. A medical history of damage to the venous system may typically include previous phlebitis, deep vein thrombosis, severe leg injury including a fracture, or varicose veins. These ulcers may take months to heal and patients are susceptible to re-ulceration at a later date.

Figure 9.5 *A venous leg ulcer showing ulceration of the gaiter area.*

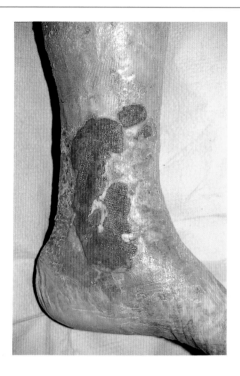

Assessment of an Ulcerated Limb

The aim of assessment is to exclude other causes of leg ulceration and to confirm a diagnosis of venous ulceration. Effective management depends on an accurate diagnosis. As only 1% of patients with leg ulceration are managed in hospital this assessment takes place either in the community or in an outpatient department (Callam *et al.* 1985).

History taking, examination and investigations form this assessment and ideally are undertaken by a multidisciplinary team.

History taking

A comprehensive medical history is taken specifically to detect venous disease and exclude other causes of ulceration (Table 9.2).

Table 9.2 *The patient's history may indicate the cause of ulceration*

Indicates venous disease	Indicates other cause of ulceration
History of:	History of:
deep vein thrombosis	diabetes (mellitus)
pulmonary embolism	vascular surgery and/or disease
previous vein surgery	intermittent claudication
fractures of the leg	rest pain
Year of first ulcer	
Number of previous episodes of ulceration	
Time this ulcer has been present	

Table 9.3 *Investigations of leg ulceration*

Investigations often undertaken	Possible further investigations
Palpation of pedal or posterior tibial pulses	Blood profiles, e.g. blood glucose level, full blood count, U & E, LFT, rheumatoid factor
Brachial blood pressure and leg systolic pressure, ankle brachial pressure index	Duplex scan
Measurement of the ulcer by tracing or photography	Venography
Measurement of ankle and leg circumference	Wound swab if infection suspected
Documentation of the ulcer site, wound bed, exudate level, previous dressings used, compression bandages used	Patch testing to determine if patient has allergies.

Examination

A physical examination is undertaken to support the medical history and to identify possible health problems which have gone unrecognized. Examination of the ulcerated limb will include:

i)   Is the shape of the leg normal, or 'champagne bottle', oedematous, or thin?

ii) Is the surrounding skin normal, smooth and well-hydrated, or eczematous, scratched, pigmented by lipodermatosclerosis or with varicose veins?

iii) Is the ankle joint fully mobile, limited mobility or completely fixed?

Investigations

The investigations listed in Table 9.3 form part of the assessment process and should not be used as the only method of determining a diagnosis.

Doppler Ultrasonographic Assessment

Doppler ultrasonography a method of measuring blood flow in peripheral arteries

i)   Make the patient comfortable. The patient should be lying flat (if possible for 20 minutes before the procedure).

ii) Locate the brachial pulse with the **Doppler ultrasonograph**, apply ultrasound gel and inflate the sphygmomanometer cuff. When the signal fades and disappears gradually deflate the cuff and record the point at which the signal returns (brachial systolic pressure).

iii) Examine the dorsal area of the ulcerated limb and locate the dorsalis pedis pulse (note that this is absent in around 12% of the population). If no pedal pulse can be located, use the posterior tibial pulse. Apply the sphygmomanometer cuff just above the ankle, warning the patient that

Figure 9.6 *Using a hand-held Doppler probe.*

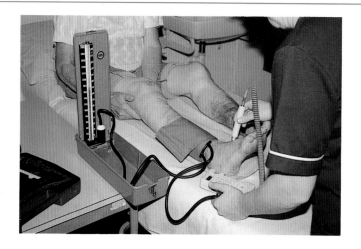

Dopplex Ankle Pressure Index (API) Guide

Ankle Pressure (mmHg)

Brachial Pressure (mmHg)	30	35	40	45	50	55	60	65	70	75	80	85	90	95	100	105	110	115	120	125	130	135	140	145	150	155	160	165	170	175	180	185	190	195	200
180	.16	.19	.22	.25	.27	.30	.33	.36	.38	.41	.44	.47	.50	.52	.55	.58	.61	.63	.66	.69	.72	.75	.77	.80	.83	.86	.89	.92	.94	.97	1.00				
175	.17	.20	.22	.25	.28	.31	.34	.37	.40	.42	.45	.48	.51	.54	.57	.60	.62	.65	.68	.71	.74	.77	.80	.82	.85	.88	.92	.94	.97	1.00					
170	.17	.20	.23	.26	.29	.32	.35	.38	.41	.44	.47	.50	.52	.55	.58	.61	.64	.67	.70	.73	.76	.79	.82	.85	.89	.91	.94	.97	1.00						
165	.18	.21	.24	.27	.30	.33	.36	.39	.42	.45	.48	.51	.54	.57	.60	.63	.66	.69	.72	.75	.78	.81	.84	.87	.90	.94	.96	1.00							
160	.18	.21	.25	.28	.31	.34	.37	.40	.43	.46	.50	.53	.56	.59	.62	.65	.68	.71	.75	.78	.81	.84	.87	.90	.93	.96	1.00								
155	.19	.22	.25	.29	.32	.35	.38	.41	.45	.48	.51	.54	.58	.61	.64	.67	.70	.74	.76	.80	.83	.87	.90	.93	.96	1.00									
150	.20	.23	.26	.30	.33	.36	.40	.43	.46	.50	.53	.56	.60	.63	.66	.70	.73	.76	.80	.83	.86	.90	.93	.96	1.00										
145	.20	.24	.27	.31	.34	.37	.41	.44	.48	.51	.55	.58	.62	.65	.69	.72	.75	.79	.82	.86	.90	.93	.96	1.00											
140	.21	.25	.28	.32	.35	.39	.42	.46	.50	.53	.57	.60	.64	.67	.71	.75	.78	.82	.85	.89	.92	.96	1.00												
135	.22	.26	.29	.33	.37	.40	.44	.48	.51	.55	.59	.62	.66	.70	.74	.77	.81	.85	.88	.92	.96	1.00													
130	.23	.27	.30	.34	.38	.42	.46	.50	.53	.57	.61	.65	.69	.73	.77	.80	.84	.88	.92	.96	1.00														
125	.24	.28	.32	.36	.40	.44	.48	.52	.56	.60	.64	.68	.72	.76	.80	.84	.88	.92	.96	1.00															
120	.25	.29	.33	.37	.40	.45	.50	.54	.58	.62	.66	.70	.75	.79	.83	.87	.91	.95	1.00																
115	.26	.30	.34	.39	.43	.48	.52	.56	.60	.65	.69	.74	.78	.82	.86	.91	.95	1.00																	
110	.27	.31	.36	.40	.45	.50	.54	.59	.63	.68	.72	.77	.81	.86	.90	.95	1.00																		
105	.28	.33	.38	.42	.47	.52	.57	.61	.66	.71	.76	.80	.85	.90	.95	1.00																			
100	.30	.35	.40	.45	.50	.55	.60	.65	.70	.75	.80	.85	.90	.95	1.00																				

GREATER THAN 1.00

HNE Diagnostics, a world leading manufacturer of pocket Dopplers, offers an extensive range of bi-directional pocket Dopplers with visual flow and rate display, together with a wide range of interchangeable probes for both vascular and obstetric applications.

WARNING: False high readings may be obtained in patients with calcified arteries because the sphygmomanometer cuff cannot fully compress the hardened arteries. Calcified arteries may be present in patients with history of Diabetes, Arteriosclerosis and Atherosclerosis.

$$\text{API} = \frac{\text{Ankle systolic pressure}}{\text{Brachial systolic pressure}}$$

Note: Diastolic pressure cannot be measured using a Doppler.

HNE
DIAGNOSTICS

Recommended Probe Frequencies:
8 MHz for normal sized limbs
5 MHz for obese / oedematous limbs

35 Portmanmoor Road, Cardiff, CF2 2HB, UK. Tel: +44 (0)1222 485885 Fax: +44 (0)1222 492520
® Dopplex, Flowtron and 'H' logo are registered trademarks of Huntleigh Technology plc in the UK, and in some cases, other territories.

A member of the Huntleigh Technology plc Group of companies. © Copyright Huntleigh Technology plc 1995   6AH239-1

Figure 9.7 *Ankle pressure index guide. (With permission of Huntleigh Healthcare, Cardiff.)*

this procedure may be uncomfortable for a few minutes. Apply ultrasound gel and inflate the cuff, listening carefully for the signal to disappear. Again, gradually deflate the cuff, noting and recording the point at which the signal returns (ankle systolic pressure) (Figure 9.6).

$$\frac{\text{ankle systolic pressure}}{\text{brachial systolic pressure}} = \text{ankle brachial pressure index}$$

A reasonable guide to using Doppler assessment (in conjunction with a full physical examination and history taking) is to use the ankle brachial pressure index (APBI) to confirm your clinical opinion (Figure 9.7). If the ABPI is considered to confirm the diagnosis, then a patient with an index of 0.8 or more will benefit from the use of compression therapy, whereas an ABPI below 0.8 is not generally considered suitable for compression.

Management

The principles of managing patients with venous ulceration lie in controlling or compensating for the damaged venous system. Although the ulcer will require a dressing, the bandaging system and compression therapy are by far the most important aspect of care. Supporting the damaged venous system using graduated compression aims to provide greater support at the ankle and less towards the knee, and is the most effective method of compensating for damaged veins (Morison and Moffatt 1994).

For patients with venous ulceration dressing materials play a far less important role than the compression bandages. Patients do find this a difficult concept to understand, focusing on the wound itself rather than the underlying pathology in the limb. Depending on assessment of the wound, any of the modern wound dressing materials may be suitable as a primary wound contact layer. The hydrophilic foams, hydrocolloids and alginates are popular, as these products can be left in place for several days at a time (Figures 9.8 to 9.12).

Graduated compression can be achieved using:

- Bandages: for maximum effectiveness compression bandages should be worn constantly when the patient is out of bed.

- Compression stockings: currently three grades of compression stocking are available in the UK, the below-knee stocking being the easiest for patients to tolerate.

- Class I stockings provide light compression of 14–17 mmHg and are used in the treatment of early varicose veins.

- Class II stockings provide more compression, 18–24 mmHg, and are used in both the treatment and prevention of venous ulceration.

- Class III stockings provide high levels of compression and are used in the prevention and treatment of patients with very large legs and also for patients with severe varicose veins.

Figure 9.8 *Tissue necrosis caused by a compression bandage applied to a leg with a poor blood supply.*

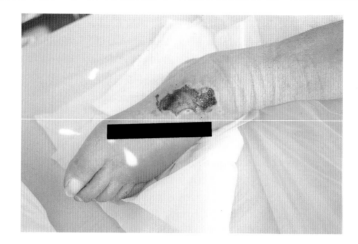

Compression stockings are fitted following measurement of the limb. It is usual for the appliance department or a trained community pharmacist to undertake fitting patients with compression stockings.

Physiotherapy

Physiotherapy may be indicated for patients who have limited mobility, limited ankle movement or fixed joints. More mobile patients should be encouraged to walk and exercise as much as possible (Figures 9.13 to 9.15). Prolonged standing should be avoided at all costs as this further impedes venous return.

Motivation and patient education

The key to success in managing patients with venous ulceration lies in involving the patient with their treatment. The nurse will provide dressings

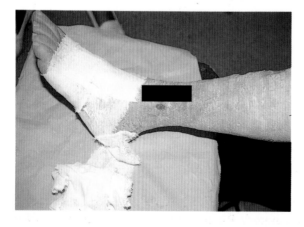

Figure 9.9 *A venous leg ulcer treated with a paste bandage. A compression bandage will be applied on top.*

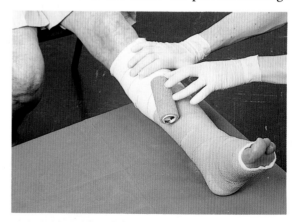

Figure 9.10 *The Charing Cross four-layer bandage system.*

Figure 9.11 *Applying bandages in a spiral arrangement. (a) Begin at the base of the toes to anchor the bandage in place. (b) Hold bandage in place with the thumb. (c) Bandage over the heel and fix with a turn around the base of the toes. (d) A view showing the inside of the foot. (e) Continue bandaging the foot using a 50% stretch. (f) Using 50% overlap continue bandaging the leg. (g) Finish at the tibial tuberosity.*

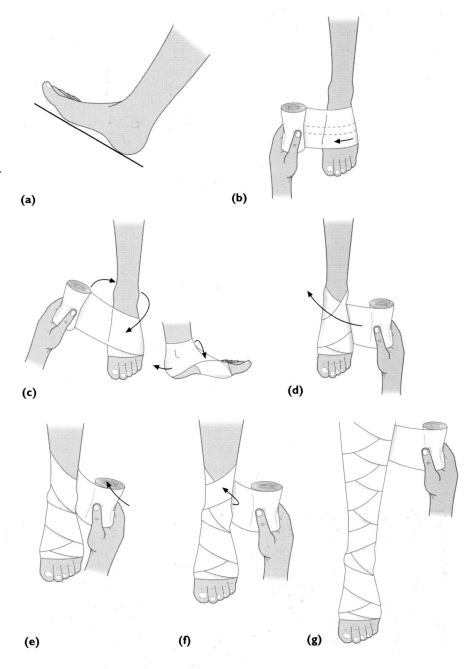

and compression, but it is the patient who is responsible for exercise and tolerance of the compression system. Patients can best help themselves if they receive appropriate information and advice and are truly integrated into their care.

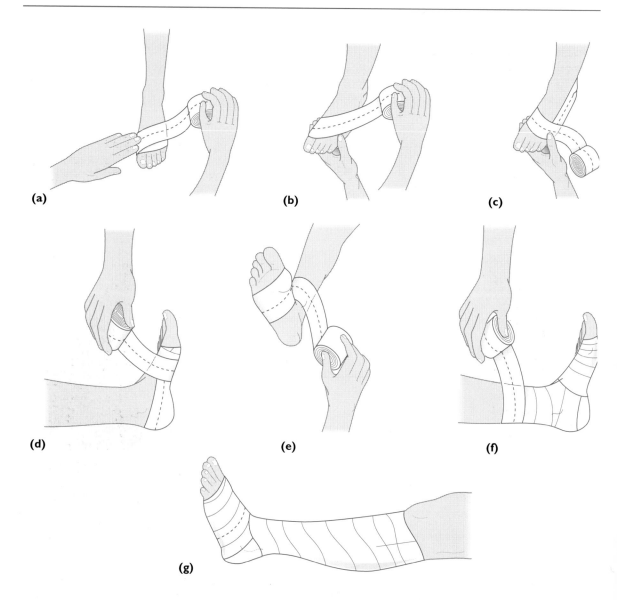

Figure 9.12 *Applying compression bandages in a figure of eight. (a) Maintain foot at a right angle to the leg. (b) Make two turns at the base of the toes. (c) Take bandage above the heel. (d) Take bandage around the heel to cover the foot. (e and f) Continue bandaging using figure of eight turns. Ensure that 50% overlap is maintained. (g) Bandage up to the tibial tuberosity.*

Nursing model for Joan

When choosing a model of care for an individual such as Joan it is important to consider the type of person the nurse is caring for. As the case study indicates, Joan is an intelligent, independent lady. She is used to telling people what to do and 'doing' for herself. Joan needs a model that focuses

Figure 9.13 *Exercises for assisting venous return: marking time while standing still.*

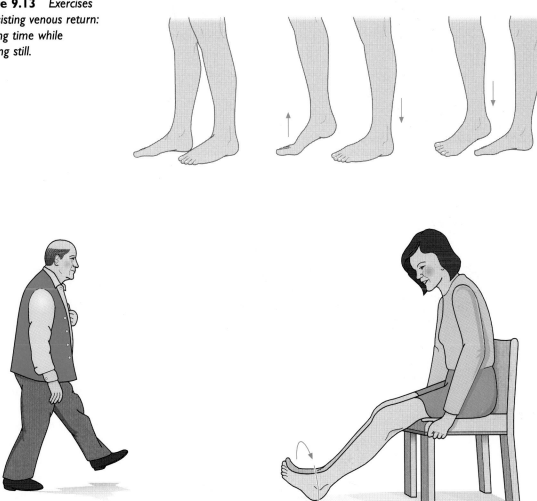

Figure 9.14 *Exercises for assisting venous return: walking as much as possible.*

Figure 9.15 *Exercises for assisting venous return: rotate ankles in a circular motion, first one way and then the other.*

on the *interaction* between nurse and patient. One that focuses on the patient's perception of the situation would be Riehl's interaction model (Riehl 1980). This model also addresses the person's interaction with their environment. Joan now has to adapt and change the way she interacts, as her normal pattern of behaviour has undergone a change. Using this model, attempt to assess Joan's problems and design a plan of care to meet her needs.

- Joan's mainstay of treatment is compression therapy. This requires both patient understanding of the treatment and compliance.
- This should not present a problem in Joan's case as long as she is treated as a true partner in care.

Arterial Ulcers

Although not as common as venous ulceration the arterial ulcer (Case Study 9.2) is considerably more problematic for patients.

Case Study 9.2 **Arterial ulcers**	Mr Jack Jones is an 83-year-old man who worked down the mines from the age of 15 years until he was 60 years old. A smoker all his life, his physical condition is poor, with frequent bouts of bronchitis during the winter due to pneumoconiosis. He lives with his wife in a small terraced house and his only social outing is a weekly visit to the servicemen's club for a game of darts.

Although the club is only at the end of the street Jack has found it increasingly difficult to get there. This is largely due to a shortage of breath but also to the cramp-like pain in his legs which increases the further he walks.

The district nurse has been treating an ulcer on the top of his right foot, where his shoe had rubbed him, for the past 18 months without any success. He now seems to have pain in his legs most of the time, even at night when the only way of relieving it is by holding his legs over the end of the bed. During the weekend Jack was only able to walk downstairs and sit in the armchair as his foot was too painful to put on the ground. On Monday morning when the nurse visited she realized the severity of his condition and called the general practitioner, who admitted him to hospital straight away.

On admission to hospital Jack was found to have a haemoglobin concentration of 9.6 g/dl and a temperature of 38.4 °C. His foot around the ulcer was red and shiny, his toes were cold to the touch. He complained of pain in the ulcer bed on touch, became very agitated when the nurse tried to dress it, and demanded a cigarette. The nurse, who was very busy and had several new admissions to the ward, replied that if he didn't stop smoking he would have to have his leg off.

Prognosis

The prognosis and outlook are often bleak if surgical intervention is not indicated. Surgical intervention can reconstruct the arteries of the lower limb, so restoring or improving the blood supply (Figure 9.16).

Figure 9.16 *(a) Arterial anatomy of a normal limb. (b) Surgical options for revascularizing the lower limb.*

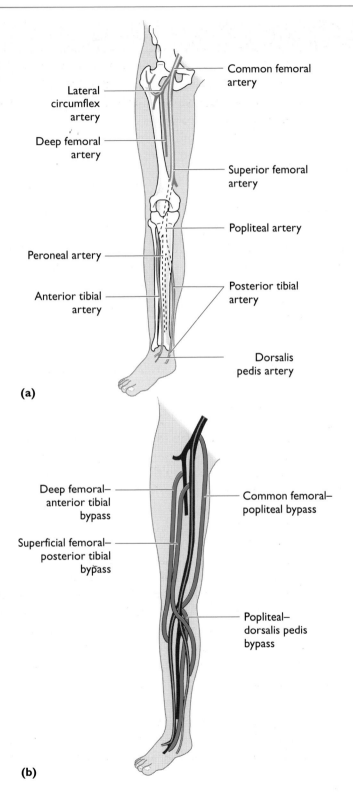

(a)

Common femoral artery

Lateral circumflex artery

Deep femoral artery

Superior femoral artery

Popliteal artery

Peroneal artery

Posterior tibial artery

Anterior tibial artery

Dorsalis pedis artery

(b)

Deep femoral–anterior tibial bypass

Common femoral–popliteal bypass

Superficial femoral–posterior tibial bypass

Popliteal–dorsalis pedis bypass

Vascular Surgery

The restoration of blood supply to the lower limb can involve a wide range of surgical procedures. For patients with isolated proximal stenotic or occlusive arterial lesions (often diabetic patients) transcutaneous balloon angioplasty is a useful, minimally invasive procedure. This procedure entails the insertion of a balloon catheter into the vascular lumen of a major artery (the iliac or femoral artery). The deflated end of the catheter is placed at the site where the stenosis occurs. When in position the balloon is inflated and stretches the vessel to enlarge the vascular lumen, so increasing blood flow distally.

Bypass surgery uses synthetic or autogenous vein grafts to replace the conduit between proximal and distal arteries, so bypassing the diseased part of the artery.

For the reconstruction of larger arteries synthetic graft material can be used as the blood flow is rapid. However, the further distally the damage, the smaller the artery involved and microsurgical techniques using an autogenous graft are preferred. Figure 9.16 shows the various options for revascularizing the lower limb.

Assessment

Assessment of the affected limb includes:

- history (typically includes night pain, relieved by holding the limb in a dependent position)
- performing a physical examination to identify perfusion and reduced body heat
- Doppler assessment to determine ABPI
- examining the wound bed particularly for the presence of devitalized tissue and infection
- identifying the presence of cellulitis related to severe infection

Patients with vascular disease require urgent referral to a vascular surgeon for a full assessment of the extent of the disease. Treatment may include angioplasty or reconstructive surgery.

Management

The principles of managing patients with arterial ulceration are control of the symptoms and observation for deterioration of either the ulcer or the limb. The prognosis for healing is poor owing to the impaired blood supply.

Local wound management

In addition to providing an optimum environment at the wound bed the nurse should be alert for deterioration in the wound bed involving tissue necrosis and the presence of wound infection. Bandages are used to retain the dressing in place and not used to provide compression.

Pain control

Pain may be a difficult problem for these patients and every effort should be made to ensure adequate and appropriate analgesia prior to dressing changes and throughout the day, as well as night sedation.

Psychological support

These patients may need a great deal of psychological support. Awareness of the problems associated with vascular disease and the possibility of losing part or all of a limb requires a sensitive approach.

Nursing model for Jack

Besides the arterial problem that makes wound healing difficult in this patient's case, the nurse has to consider a model that will enlist the patient's cooperation otherwise he will not comply with any of the suggested treatments. Unfortunately his hospital admission did not set off on the right footing and much skill will be required to enlist the patient's trust in the staff and the system. Peplau's model emphasizes the interpersonal relationship between the nurse and patient and how it must develop in order for the patient's condition to improve.

The developmental models emphasize re-establishment of a developmental stage from which the individual has regressed. Intervention in these models often focuses on the educative–counselling role of the nurse which is likely to be of more importance in this case than actual treatment of the ulcer. Using Peplau's SOAP structure, try to identify a plan of care; for example:

S — complains of pain in his calf and foot
     has no appetite for food
     desperate for cigarettes
O — ulcer bed red and bleeding to touch
     area around ulcer erythematous
     looks pale and thin
     troublesome cough
A — ulcer showing clinical signs of infection
     temperature 38.4 °C
     haemoglobin level 9.6 g/dl
     pneumoconiosis exacerbated by smoking 20–25 cigarettes a day
P — goal is eradication of infection
     take swab to identify infecting organism
     prescribe appropriate systemic antibiotics

Practice points

- As Jack has an infection that needs to be treated, the problems initially identified are those of a physical nature. This is in line with Peplau's philosophy that the first purpose of the nurse is to help the patient to survive. The nurse can also make a significant difference to the amount of pain Jack is experiencing if the infection is treated correctly. This can form a basis on which a trusting relationship can develop. However, to build upon the nurse–patient relationship, it is essential to identify the psychosocial problems.
- Maybe the nurse voiced Jack's underlying fear, i.e. that of losing his leg.
- Continue working on this care plan, identifying problems and goals and planning the appropriate care.

Fungating Malignant Wounds

The psychological problems of fungating malignant lesions, as described in Case Study 9.3, can be as great as the physical problems.

Case Study 9.3
Fungating malignant wounds

Mrs Dorothy Phillips is a 73-year-old retired nurse who was admitted to a hospice for management of a fungating carcinoma of her left breast. Although aware of changes in the shape of her breast some 4 years ago, Dorothy choose to ignore it until finally, prompted by her husband, she went to her general practitioner a year ago. By this time she was having discharge from the nipple and the surrounding skin had the characteristic *peau d'orange* (orange peel) appearance. As Dorothy and her worried husband had feared, she had a large tumour underneath her nipple which had progressed so extensively that surgery was not recommended. Following a short course of chemotherapy and radiotherapy both Mr and Mrs Phillips and her oncologist decided that aggressive treatment was too physically and mentally distressing and that she would prefer palliative treatment only.

On admission to the hospice Dorothy was found to have the whole area of the left breast covered with fungating, malodorous, sloughy tissue. The malignancy had extended throughout the breast and into the lymphatic system, causing extensive lymphoedema of her left arm and leaving it immobilized.

Dorothy was fairly cheerful, although tired and anxious to return home as soon as possible. She was aware of her prognosis, but was reluctant to discuss it openly. She was very distressed by advancing disease so evident in the wound. The odour was upsetting her and she was anxious that something could be done to keep the smell at bay, as she was embarrassed when visitors came to call. While she was at home her husband had, with the district nurse's assistance, been dressing the wound, but it now required changing three or four times a day due to the constant leakage of exudate. She was not in any undue pain from the tumour, but was becoming increasingly short of breath due to secondary deposits in her lung.

Aetiology

The incidence of fungating and ulcerating lesions is most commonly associated with breast cancer in women (Figure 9.17) although there is little documentation with regard to the prevalence in recent years.

Common sites for ulceration include maligant melanoma, carcinoma of the oral cavity (Rosen 1980), head and neck, uterus, cervix, vagina and vulva (Charles-Edwards 1983). Thomas (1992) identified the percentage and location of fungating wounds that were treated by specialist centres as shown in Table 9.4.

Lesions infiltrate the epithelium and supporting lymph and blood vessels and, as the tumour extends, capillaries rupture leading to tissue breakdown and necrosis. Fungating malignant lesions occur when there is cancerous infiltration of the epithelium resulting in ulceration through the skin to the body surface (Dealey 1994). The cause is usually:

- an undiagnosed or ignored primary tumour or recurrence after surgery, radiotherapy or chemotherapy (Petrek *et al.* 1983)
- a rapidly progressing, aggressive tumour (Rosen 1980)

Often the lesion presents as a foul-smelling fungating mass, owing to colonization by anaerobic organisms.

Management

Improvement in the quality of life of patient and family can be achieved by alleviating the distressing symptoms of pain, infection, bleeding, malodour and discharge. Above all, it is essential to maintain the patient's dignity and

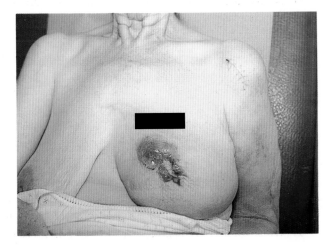

Figure 9.17 *A fungating malignant tumour of the left breast.*

Table 9.4 *Wound location in patients with fungating tumours undergoing treatment in specialist centres*

Location of wound	Percentage of total
Breast	62
Head/face	24
Groin/genitals	3
Back	3
Others	8

From Thomas (1992).

self-esteem. One can support carers and patient in care of the lesion by adopting a positive outlook to management. Patients may be considered incurable once skin ulceration is present, even without metastases. Twenty-four out of 38 patients died within 1 year in Petrek's study (Petrek *et al.* 1983), although Sims and Fitzgerald (1985) reported survival of longer than 2 years despite extensive lesions. When treatment with curative intent is no longer appropriate or effective, carers must attempt to improve the quality of life and adopt a positive approach to topical management of the lesion.

Radiotherapy

Wound assessment should also include the potential for radiotherapy, which can decrease tumour bulk and exudate, in turn decreasing pain. It also allows some healing at the margins when the tumour bulk has decreased.

Wound management

The practitioner's attitude, especially during dressing procedures, can greatly influence the patient's own attitude and acceptance of the disease (Charles-Edwards 1983).

Whereas physical symptoms can be controlled, the psychological effects of the pressure of advancing disease can be intensely distressing to patients, carers and relatives (Wells 1984). Feelings may range from depression, shame and embarrassment, to rejection and revulsion.

Cleansing fungating and ulcerating wounds with antiseptics was widely thought to inhibit bacterial proliferation and diminish the offensive smell of anaerobic infection. Generally this has been found to be ineffective, as most cleansing agents are inactivated by body fluids (Leaper *et al.* 1987) and, in some cases, can cause damage to new tissue (Leaper 1986). As bleeding points can be easily disturbed, only gentle irrigation with warm water or saline should be undertaken to remove debris and old dressings.

Topical metronidazole is effective in reducing odour (Newman *et al.* 1989, Bower *et al.* 1992), and can be applied directly onto the fungating mass and covered. Alternatively, it can be used in conjunction with an amorphous hydrogel which will provide greater absorbency (Dealey 1994). Topical metronidazole is particularly useful for controlling malodour in malignant fungating lesions as anaerobic organisms, usually *Bacteroides*, colonize these lesions (Thomas 1989).

Dressings

Grocott (1992) identified the following principles that can be applied to the management of any fungating wound:

- The control of pain through maintenance of optimum humidity at the wound site by using dressings that do not adhere to the tumour
- Facilitation of wound debridement with removal of excess exudate and toxic materials to prevent deterioration and control smell
- Topical antibiotics to control odour when appropriate
- Removal of dressings without trauma
- Restoration of body symmetry through use of cavity dressings
- Achievement of cosmetic acceptability, without the need for bulky secondary dressings
- Control bleeding when it occurs by using haemostatic dressings

Nursing model for Dorothy

Roy's adaptation model (Roy 1980) has been described in other works (Chadderton 1986) and is a useful framework when nursing the terminally ill. As outlined in Chapter 6, Roy's model is consistent with the hospice philosophy, in that when active treatment is not possible, symptomatic relief will help patients adapt to their particular situations and allow them to come to terms with their illness. Try using this model to plan the care for Dorothy.

Practice points

Dorothy Phillips may (unlike Fiona Starr in Chapter 6) have adapted to her situation, although denial has been a major part of her response to her illness. With the visible advancement of her disease both she and her husband may need to adapt to this stimulus in a way that will give them an improved quality of life in the terminal stages.

Summary

This chapter illustrates the importance of the nurse–patient relationship whether it concerns helping a patient to understand the nature of their wound, or coming to terms with disfigurement. What important features do these clinical case studies highlight for the nurse to consider?

- Educator — helping the patient with venous disease understand the importance of compression therapy in the healing process

- Counsellor — giving the patient with arterial disease the opportunity to express their fears regarding their disease process

- Advocate — maintaining the dignity and self-esteem of the patient with fungating wounds

Once you are familiar with these basic principles of wound management, the above roles will enable you to enhance your care to a higher level of specialism.

Further Reading

Kulozik M, Cherry GW & Ryan TJ (1986) The importance of measuring the ankle/brachial systolic pressure ratio in the management of leg ulcers. *British Journal of Dermatology* 115(Suppl): 26–27.

Stami SK, Shields JH, Sairr JH & Coleridge Smith PD (1992) Leg ulceration in venous disease. *Postgraduate Medical Journal* 68: 779–785.

Callam MJ, Harper DR, Dale JJ & Ruckley CV (1987) Arterial disease in chronic leg ulceration: an under estimated hazard? Lothian and Forth Valley leg ulcer study. *British Medical Journal* 294: 929–931.

Negus D (1992) *Leg Ulcers. A Practical Approach to Management.* Oxford: Butterworth-Heinemann.

Ruckley CV (1988) *A Colour Atlas of Surgical Management of Venous Disease.* London: Wolfe.

Ryan T (1992) *The Management of Leg Ulcers* 2nd edn. Oxford University Press.

Dodd H & Cockett FB (eds) (1976) The pathology and surgery of veins of the lower limb, 2nd edn. Edinburgh: Churchill Livingstone.

Foltz A (1980) Fungating and ulcerating malignant lesions: A review of the literature. *Journal of Advanced Nursing* 7(2): 8–13.

Morison M & Moffatt C (1994) *A Colour Guide to the Assessment and Management of Leg Ulcers.* 2nd edn. London: Mosby.

Boulton AJM, Connor H & Cavanagh PR (1994) *The Foot in Diabetes.* 2nd edn. Chichester: Wiley.

References

Bower M, Stein R, Evans TRJ, Hedley A, Pett P & Coombes RC (1992) A double blind study of the efficacy of Metronidazole gel in the treatment of malodorous fungating tumours. *European Journal of Cancer* 28A: 415; 888–889.

Callam MJ, Ruckley CV, Harper DR & Dale JJ (1985) Chronic ulceration of the leg: extent of the problem and provision of care. *British Medical Journal* 290: 1855–1856.

Callam MJ, Harper DR, Dale JJ & Ruckley CV (1987) Chronic ulceration of the leg: clinical history. Lothian and Forth Valley Leg Ulcer Study.

Chadderton H (1986) A stress adaptation model in terminal care. In: Kershaw B & Salvage J (eds) *Models for Nursing*. Chichester: Wiley.

Charles-Edwards A (1983) *The nursing care of the dying patient*. Beaconfield: Beaconfield Ltd.

Dealey C (1994) A problem solving approach to wound care. *Journal of Community Nursing* 8: 8.

Fletcher A (1992) The epidemiology of two common age-related wounds. *Journal of Wound Care* 1(4): 39–43.

Grocott P (1992) Application of the principles of modern wound management for complex wounds. *Palliative Care*. In: Proceedings of the First European Conference on Advances in Wound Management. London: Macmillan.

Leaper D (1986) Antiseptics and their effect on healing tissue. *Nursing Times* 83(22): 45–47.

Leaper D, Cameron S & Lancaster J (1987) Antiseptic solutions. *Community Outlook* 83(14): 30–34.

Morison M & Moffatt C (1994) *A Colour Guide to the Assessment and Management of Leg Ulcers*. 2nd edn. London: Mosby.

Newman V, Allwood M & Oakes RA (1989) THe use of Metronidazole gel to control the smell of malodour. *Palliative Medicine* 3: 303–305.

Petrek JA, Glenn PD & Cramer AR (1983) Ulcerated breast cancer: patients and outcome. *American Surgeon* 49(4): 187–191.

Riehl JP (1980) The Riehl interaction model. In: Riehl JP & Roy C (eds) *Conceptual Models for Nursing Practice*. New York: Appleton-Century-Crofts.

Roy C (1980) The Roy adaptation model. In: Riehl JP & Roy C (eds) *Conceptual Models for Nursing Practice*. New York: Appleton-Century-Crofts.

Rosen T (1980) Cutaneous metastases. *Medical Clinics of North America* 64(5): 885–900.

Sims R & Fitzgerald V (1985) Community Nursing. Management of Patients with Ulcerating/Fungating Malignant Breast Disease. London: RCN Oncology Nursing Society.

Thomas S (1989) Treating malodorous wounds. *Community Outlook* Oct: 27–30.

Thomas S (1992) *Current practices in the management of fungating lesions and radiation damaged skin*. Surgical Materials Testing Laboratory, Bridgend General Hospital, Mid-Glamorgan.

Wells R (1984) Wound care. Clinical Forum. *Nursing Mirror* 158: 10–15.

Wilson E (1989) Prevention and treatment of venous leg ulcers. *Health Trends* 4: 21–97.

EVALUATION

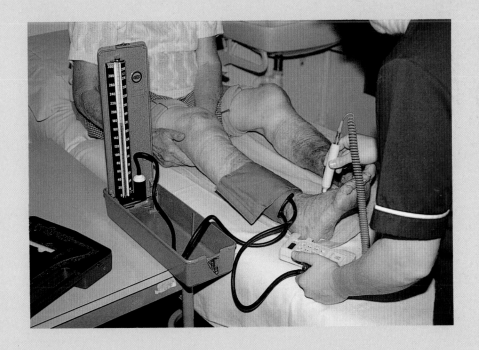

10 Ways of Evaluating Care

Key issues

This chapter outlines different ways in which patient care can be measured and evaluated. Four main areas are considered:

■ Evaluation of the wound:
  wound measurement techniques

■ Evaluation of the delivery of care:
  audit
  standard setting
  use of protocols and guidelines

■ Evaluation of the patient:
  quality of life research

■ Evaluation of the nurse:
  role of the nurse specialist

Introduction

With increasing demands from the government and the general public for successful and measurable outcomes, methods of evaluating care are now a central focus of modern wound management.

The methods of evaluation will depend on what is being evaluated. It is easy to evaluate if a wound has healed when skin integrity is achieved, but emotional healing of a wound caused by a burn or similar traumatic injury will be difficult to quantify. Interest is now being expressed in the patients' quality of life, especially for patients living with chronic wounds such as leg ulcers. Wound measurement on a regular basis can determine the rate of healing and can be used to evaluate if progress is being achieved according to the plan of management.

As outlined earlier, goals and outcomes should be set with evaluation in mind; use of subjective terminology will be difficult to evaluate and tells us nothing about the patient's care.

Evaluation of the Wound

Wound measurement techniques can be divided into contact and non-contact methods (Table 10.1). For the majority of nurses in everyday practice the simplest and easiest way of measuring the wound progress is

Table 10.1 *Wound measurement techniques*

Contact	Non-contact
Tracing overlays	Structured light
Depth gauges	Laser triangulation
Moulding material	Photogrammetry
Liquids	Stereophotogrammetry
Surface contour tracings	Monte Carlo technique
Ultrasound	Magnetic resonance imaging

From Melhuish *et al.* (1994).

the use of contact measurements. Tracing overlays, depth gauges or surface contour tracings are used (Figure 10.1).

Other methods such as filling the wound with saline to compare the amount of liquid the wound holds on each occasion (Berg *et al.* 1990) or

Figure 10.1 *Kundig gauge. Reproduced with permission from Kundin JI (1989) American Journal of Nursing* **2***: 206–207.*

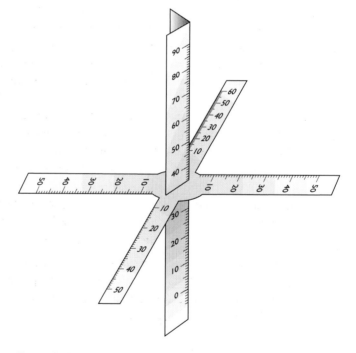

Formula I: Area of Surface Lesion
Step 1. N + S = value A
Step 2. E + W = value B
Step 3. Multiply (A x B) by **.785** to find the **area**.

Formula II: Volume of Crater Wound
Step 1. N + S = value A
Step 2. E + W = value B
Step 3. Depth reading of vertical axis = value C
Step 4. Multiply (A x B x C) by **.327** to find the **volume**.

using dental moulding material (Resch *et al.* 1988) are time-consuming and generally not suited to everyday practice. However, contact measurements tend to be unreliable as they give only a two-dimensional reading. They also have the disadvantage of the risk of wound contamination, and often discrepancies between measurement of the same wound have been observed when different nurses are taking readings (Anthony 1993).

Non-contact methods that give three-dimensional readings are proving to be a more sensitive measure of both area and volume, and techniques such as structured light measurement (Plassman and Jones 1992), which gives an accurate picture of wound depth, are exciting new developments.

The relationship between wound area, volume and circumference has been demonstrated in various studies (Eriksson *et al.* 1979; Bulstrode *et al.* 1987; Melhuish *et al.* 1994). It remains a matter of debate, however, as to which is the best predictor of healing: area and circumference, volume and circumference, or all three together.

Non-contact techniques such as these are the way forward as they provide accurate and objective wound measurement and therefore better evaluation of healing, or non-healing. However, these complex measures are not yet available to most practitioners, and the simpler contact measurements — although less reliable — are at present the best choice available.

Evaluating Quality of Care

In order to maintain or improve the quality of care the patient receives, nursing care needs to be measured and evaluated. How can we be assured that the quality of care is being maintained, or even reached at all?

Quality can be evaluated in one of two ways (Morison 1992):

- By taking a systematic look at practice, reviewing the results within a peer group, identifying problems and possible solutions, and implementing change — this is known as the audit cycle
- By setting a standard that individuals, teams, organizations can agree upon, monitoring that standard, having a peer group review, identifying the problems if any, and implementing changes as required — this is known as the standard setting cycle

Audit

Audit involves taking a systematic look at practice, which may be done at random without any change in practice being made, or linked to standard-setting where criteria relating to the standard can be measured in the audit (Figure 10.2).

Clinical audit has been defined by the Department of Health (1993) as a 'systematic look at the procedures used for diagnosis, care and treatment, examining how associated resources are used and investigating the effect care has on the outcome and quality of life for the patient'. Ideally audit should be multidisciplinary, but in general it is carried out by doctors and nurses. It

Figure 10.2 *Audit.*
(From Morison 1992.)

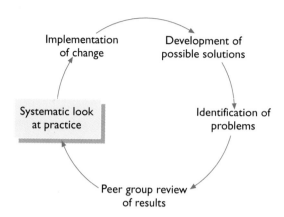

should focus on the patient, aiming to improve clinical effectiveness and therefore the quality of care the patient receives. Audits can be carried out retrospectively after care has been given, or prospectively while the patient is being cared for.

Various methods of auditing can be used depending on the professional focus, but questionnaires, interviews or examination of nursing notes and medical records may be used. There are various 'ready-made' nursing audit tools such as Monitor or Qualpacs which have been used in a variety of settings and provide a useful starting point for nurses to examine the quality of care (Harvey 1988). Audit can be carried out informally at ward or health clinic level, or formally at unit or directorate level.

Standard Setting

Why set standards?

Setting standards can help to provide an acceptable level of care to patients and carers. Considered to be part of a package that leads to quality, standards can be used as a means of evaluating the level of care given. Standard setting is a dynamic process (Figure 10.3).

How do we know that the standards set are acceptable to our patients and to other colleagues? Everybody has individual standards. Standards that we set ourselves, and on which we base the way we live, will have been largely influenced by our cultural and environmental background, but, as with the standard-setting cycle, these will change and develop according to influences around us in everyday life.

Certain standards within a professional organization such as nursing will have been set, and nurses are expected to conform to them on becoming part of the profession, but even these standards change according to the social and cultural norms of the environment. For example, it was standard practice in nursing in the 1970s to address patients by their surname and title (Mrs,

Figure 10.3 *Standard-setting cycle. (From Morison 1992.)*

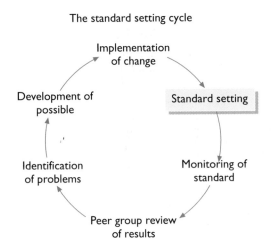

The standard setting cycle

Implementation
of change

Standard setting

Development of
possible

Monitoring of
standard

Identification
of problems

Peer group review
of results

Mr, etc.) and to refer to colleagues as 'Sister', 'Staff Nurse' or 'Doctor'. This practice reflected aspects of life outside nursing. This standard has now changed to a less formal approach, with patients and staff often calling each other by their first names. This may be seen by some as a lowering of standards, especially for nurses who trained in the era when last names only were used. This is a subjective type of standard which refers to a person's attitude or belief and is difficult to measure whether it affects the quality of care given.

Standards that directly affect the level of care given are concerned with knowledge and skills. For example, it is generally accepted that inadequate hand-washing is a major source of cross-infection and leads to a higher incidence of wound infection. A hospital may have set a standard such as 'post-operative wound infection will be no higher than 5%'. Nurses may accept this as a hospital standard, but lack the knowledge of the mechanisms of cross-infection or the skills of performing adequate hand-washing. It is therefore of vital importance that these things are considered when standards are set, otherwise they will not be achieved. Because there will always be different perspectives from nurses, doctors, patients and the organization, it is often difficult to set an acceptable standard.

Advantages of setting standards

Written standards allow practice to be critically examined. It is a way of bringing theory and practice together and highlights where resources, knowledge and skills are lacking.

As in the example of cross-examination and wound infection given above, it could be assumed that all nurses know about correct hand-washing technique and its role in prevention of post-operative infection. However, it was only when this standard statement was formulated that these two key factors were addressed by the introduction of an educational programme on infection control.

Standard setting gives nurses and other professionals an opportunity to ask what they are trying to achieve and if they achieve it.

Disadvantages of setting standards

Standards are often accused of being a statement of the obvious and are seen as a paper exercise. Many practitioners do not see the benefit of written standards as they are convinced that their personal standard of care is good enough and that they maintain a consistently high standard of care at all times. This may well be true of many individuals involved in providing care, but there is no proof to support this belief and they may be totally ignorant of the potential harm this practice may cause.

Standards are difficult to formulate for reasons already discussed. The process is time-consuming, it is often difficult to get people together and, initially difficulty may be experienced in choosing a topic or problem through which to develop a standard (Johns 1989). However, all these problems are surmountable and once the commitment from the participants is there, the process can be stimulating and rewarding (Johns 1989).

How to write standards for wound care

Ideally standards of care should be set and written by members of an interprofessional team. This avoids potential conflicts of interest between team members and provides a holistic approach to patient care (Wright and Whittington 1992).

The most widely used framework for writing standards is that of Donabedian (1976) using the criteria of structure, process and outcome. Following formulation of a standard statement, these three criteria describe how and whether the standard is being achieved:

- *Structure* involves the resources used to provide care and the manner in which they are organized
- *Process* is the way in which the professionals and others use the resources and the manner in which care is given
- *Outcome* is the end result in terms of health and client satisfaction

The standard *statement* is the broad objective of the standard which specifies the level of quality, for example

'All patients must receive information regarding clinic delays'

Indicators of whether or not this standard can be and is being achieved are found in the criteria. They need to be relevant, understandable, measurable, behavioural and achievable (Marr and Giebing 1994):

- *Relevant* to the activity to which they are applied
- *Understandable* by *all* those working in the area
- *Measurable* with the *minimum* amount of effort, time and resources
- *Flexible* so that criteria can be changed according to service and client need
- *Locally owned* (but written in accordance with management standards)

Not all standards will be written using this outline of structure, process and outcome. Some will have a standard statement followed by a list of criteria (Hopper 1991).

Formulation of criteria will be based on professional experience, values and beliefs, legal requirements, policies and guidelines for practice that are in use in the area for which standards are being set. The set standards and criteria must always fit in with the aims of the organization and existing statutes of governing bodies (Marr and Giebing 1994).

It is equally important to ensure that, once the standard has been written, a review date is set.

Protocols and Guidelines

While setting standards is a method of evaluating the quality of patient care, the use of protocols and guidelines can further enhance quality assurance by providing the practitioner with a rational, research-based method of managing wounds.

Nursing still abounds with ritualistic practice, which is often not justified by current research (Walsh and Ford 1989), and with the rapid expansion in wound care products it is often easier to stick to what has always been done rather than change to a new method of care.

Although nurses remain largely responsible for changing dressings, there continues to be conflict between doctor and nurse as to who should make the decision regarding the type of dressings to be used. Gwyther (1988) found that 83.5% of nurses stated that a sister or staff nurse made this decision, whereas 45.9% felt that it also could be the doctor. (Percentage totals over 100 due to multiple responses.) Flanagan (1992) revealed that nurses choose dressings for pressure sores, but surgeons generally had a larger input in care of surgical wounds.

Rapid expansion of the development of sophisticated dressings means that unit costs of dressings also rise, and decision-making may be dictated by this rather than by appropriate research-based evidence. With all of these factors to consider, many health authorities have realized the benefit of producing wound care protocols which are linked to hospital formularies.

What is the difference between a protocol and guideline?

Protocols are generally considered to be more rigid and less flexible in their approach. They may often be based on national or international research findings and have legal implications for a practitioner who does not follow them, e.g. protocols that have been developed by doctors and nurses in primary health teams for asthma or diabetic clinics will have been approved by the governing Family Health Services Authority. Often both guidelines and protocols will be linked to local health authority/trusts policies or guidelines.

Guideline is a less binding framework within which the practitioners can follow their own code of professional conduct. An example of guidelines for acute wound management is given in the Appendix.

Despite the differences between protocols and guidelines, the advantages and disadvantages of writing and using them are similar.

Advantages of protocols and guidelines

- Wound management is a fast-growing speciality — should keep abreast of new treatments
- Based on research findings
- Provides a systematic framework within which practitioners can practise confidently and safely
- Ensures continuity of care
- Discourages the use of individual preferences and 'ritualistic' practice
- Brings team members together during production of the document
- Offers a basis for evaluation of care through audit
- Maximizes cost-effective care when linked to hospital formulary

Disadvantages of protocols and guidelines

- Require a team approach to ensure broad aspect
- Difficult to get people together as a team
- Take time to set up and write
- Difficult to disseminate especially if not adopted at local level (Russell and Grimshaw 1992)
- Need piloting to be successful
- Legal aspects of protocols especially if linked to performance criteria of job description
- Problems of convincing practitioners they need them
- Need to be constantly reviewed and updated to remain current

All the above methods tell us about the care we give as nurses in terms of objective, measurable outcomes. The traditional evaluation of medical or nursing treatments has been through quantitative measurements of healing rates or reduction in morbidity. An area that has been ignored until recently is how the patient feels, and what psychosocial problems affect the patient's day-to-day living. Quality of life research is now directed at trying to quantify the subjective experiences of these patients.

Evaluating the Patient's Quality of Life

The term 'quality of life' is often used freely among health professionals with the assumption that everybody has the same understanding of what it refers to.

Quality of life is such a broad concept and is so subjective that many clinicians still question its relevance or validity to a patient's outcome. Indeed, all nurses would like to think that they are able to improve their patients' quality of life by maintaining a good standard of nursing care.

As previously outlined, standards of care vary between individuals, as does the definition of what constitutes a good quality of life. Although quality of life outcomes are a move away from the traditional medical outcomes, definitions are still largely concerned with health-related outcomes; for example, Fallowfield (1990), a psychologist, defined four areas or core domains, of which psychological factors were placed first.

- Psychological:
    depression
    anxiety
    adjustment or illness
- Social:
    Personal and sexual relationships
    Engagement in social and leisure activities
- Occupational:
    ability and desire to carry out paid employment
    ability to cope with household duties
- Physical:
    pain
    mobility
    sleep
    appetite and nausea
    sexual functioning

The order of these core domains may be rearranged according to the individual's professional background, e.g. a nurse may list the physical or social domain as being of greater importance, whereas a social worker would probably consider occupational needs.

Todd (1992) listed only three areas for evaluation:

- Physical:
    pain
    mobility
    sleep
    appetite and nausea
    sexual functioning
- Psychological:
    depression

anxiety
adjustment or illness
- Social:
personal and sexual relationships
engagement in social and leisure activities

It can be argued that nurses have already identified these as important aspects of a patient's overall quality of life, given that most nursing models address these core areas in their assessment framework. However, having identified these problem areas in the nursing assessment, how can they be evaluated to demonstrate a significant improvement to the patient's quality of life?

As it is such a difficult area to define and measure, researchers have attempted to create standardized tests using a psychometric approach (Price *et al.* 1994).

Psychometric Tests

Psychometry uses standardized tests to measure any given concept (Price *et al.* 1993). There are several tests in use, which are either generic or disease-specific. Generic tests cover a wide range of domains, the most widely used being the Nottingham Health Profile (Hunt *et al.* 1989) and the SF-36 Health Survey (see Appendix).

Disease-specific tools have been designed for various disorders such as diabetes mellitus (Wallymahmed *et al.* 1991) and chronic pain (Chibnall and Tait 1990). The decision as to which test will evaluate effectively the patient's quality of life will depend on the type of patient and wound under study and the particular research or clinical questions that need to be answered. There is probably, at present, no test that adequately measures those suffering from long-term wounds.

Previous authors have used a variety of established tests together to investigate quality of life in patients with leg ulcers (Hamer *et al.* 1994). Price *et al.* (1994) however, designed a specific questionnaire based on specialist opinions of the relevant domains important to patients with acute surgical cavity wounds.

Look at the examples of the Nottingham Health Profile and the SF-36 in the Appendix. Which particular domains of these tests do you see as being important measures of quality of life for a patient for whom you are currently caring?

Evaluating the Contribution of the Specialist Nurse

So far we have looked at ways of evaluating the progress of the wound, the quality of care given, or the quality of life of the patient. Perhaps, finally, it is appropriate to look at the role of specialist nurses and evaluate their unique skills that can influence the overall care and management of the patient.

The Clinical Nurse Specialist

Hamric and Spross (1989) defined the Clinical Nurse Specialist as 'a registered nurse who, through study and supervised practice at a graduate level has become an expert in a defined area of knowledge and practice in a selected clinical area of nursing'. Although there are many nurses who call themselves Clinical Nurse Specialists (CNS) in the UK, there is at present no formal education pathway to follow.

In wound care, the role of the CNS can vary greatly, from tissue viability nurses, whose main area of specialism is centred around pressure sore prevention, to leg ulcer specialists. Because of the disparity in roles it is often difficult to evaluate how effective these specialists are, and they are often the target of criticism by the generalist nurse. Accused of being protective of their special skills and knowledge in order to retain power (Chapman 1983), the CNS is said to know more and more about less and less (Wade and Moyer 1989).

In an era where holism and primary nursing are underpinning practices, the increasing number of specialists who may care for one patient can be construed as promoting the reductionist approach so strongly criticized in medicine. Humphris (1994) refers to this problem as 'task allocation by another name'.

The CNS has five commonly accepted major roles (Storr 1988):

- Practitioner — carries out direct patient care
- Teacher and educator — to patient, family, nursing staff, students
- Consultant — plans and advises on total care with patient, family, nursing staff
- Researcher — carries out research relevant to speciality
- Change agent — acts as catalyst for change within the organization

Consider these five roles in relation to a nurse specialist in wound care.

Practitioner

In carrying out direct patient care the CNS can act as a role model for other practitioners with whom they are in contact.

Using their advanced knowledge of wound care they are able to assess patients comprehensively using a nursing model where appropriate, while developing individual nursing care plans.

Their advanced nursing skills enable care to be delivered at a high level, setting the standard to be followed by those continuing the day-to-day nursing care of the patient.

Teacher and educator

Wound care specialists can disseminate knowledge among other practitioners, patients and carers in the clinical application of their work. Often they are responsible for setting up courses (Flanagan 1995, Jones 1995), clinics and link-nurse schemes. Professional groups such as the Tissue Viability Society and Wound Care Society which are run and supported by specialist nurses also contribute to the spread of knowledge as they provide peer support, organize study days, and produce newsletters and journals.

Consultant

Psychological support of staff and patients is an essential aspect of the role of the CNS (Dealey 1990). Often specialists will act as counsellors for staff and patients as they are seen as being approachable (Fenton 1985). It is vitally important, therefore, that individuals undertaking this role are easily accessible to both staff and patients.

Researcher

A major part of the specialist role is involvement in research. Conducting research trials or evaluating existing research constitutes a large part of the day-to-day work of the CNS. Nurses are often accused of not reading current research or transferring research findings into practice; the specialist can bridge this gap between theory and practice to the benefit of both nurse and patient.

Change agent

The specialist should act as a catalyst for change within the organization. However, change is often difficult to achieve, but the specialist can overcome resistance by using communication skills and fostering relationships with medical and nursing staff. Seen to occupy a position of power and often viewed as having charismatic qualities (Storr 1988), the specialist can change ritualistic and outdated practices which are often detrimental to patient care (Flanagan 1992).

The benefits of specialist nursing

The above roles illustrate the qualities the wound care specialist is required to have and how they can be used in practice. Research has confirmed that expertise, further training and effective methods of organizing care are essential components of quality patient care (Centre for Health Economics 1992).

Where the CNS is perceived as a powerful clinical expert and is an accepted figure in the organization in which the CNS is employed, then high-quality nursing practice is seen to be the result (Sparacino 1986).

Wound care specialists are increasing in number, as is the level of education available to them. To obtain a true evaluation of their effectiveness on the quality of care, further research will be required.

Practice point

- If you work with wound care specialists think of ways in which they improve the quality of care the patient receives

Summary

Evaluation of care can be achieved in many different ways. Each method concentrates on a particular aspect of wound care.

Evaluation should always be considered at the assessment and planning phase of management, not as an afterthought.

The main areas of evaluation can be summarized as follows:

- evaluation of the wound:
    wound measurement techniques
- evaluation of the delivery of care:
    audit
    standard setting
    protocols or guidelines
- evaluation of the patient:
    quality of life
- evaluation of the nurse
    role of the specialist nurse in wound care

Further Reading   Hirokawa RY (1986) *Communication and Group Decision-making*. Beverley Hills, Ca: Sage.

Hamric AB & Spross J (eds) (1983) *The Clinical Nurse Specialist in Theory and Practice*. New York: Grune & Stratton.

Flanagan M (1992) The role of the specialist nurse in wound care. *Journal of Wound Care* 1(2): 45–46.

Lock S & Wells F (eds) (1993) *Fraud and Misconduct in Medical Research*. London: BMJ Publishing.

Bowling A (1991) *Measuring Health: A Review of Quality of Life Measurement Scales*. Oxford University Press.

Lindholm C, Bjellerup M, Christensen OB & Zederfelt B (1994) Quality of life in chronic leg ulcer patients: an assessment according to the Nottingham Health Profile. *Proceedings of the Third European Conference on Advances in Wound Management*. London: Macmillan.

National Organisation of Quality Assurances in Hospitals (1992). Quality Assurance in European Hospitals: Results of the assessment phase of a concerted action programme covering 262 hospitals in 15 countries. Utrecht: National Organisation for Quality Assurance in Hospitals.

Kitson AL (1989) *Standards of Care. A Framework for Quality*. London: Scutari.

Luthert JM & Robinson L (eds) (1993) *The Royal Marsden Hospital manual of standards of care*. Oxford: Blackwell.

Melhuish JM, Plassman P & Harding KG (1994) Circumference, area and volume of the healing wound. *Journal of Wound Care* 3(8): 380–384.

Majeske C (1992) Reliability of wound surface area measurements. *Physical Therapy* 72: 138–141.

Bernett G & Moody M (1995) *Wound Care for Health Professionals*. London: Chapman & Hall.

References

Anthony D (1993) Measuring pressure sores and venous leg ulcers. *Community Outlook* August, 35–36.

Berg W, Traneroth C, Gunnarsson A & Lossing C (1990) A method for measuring pressure sores. *Lancet* 335: 1445–1446.

Bulstrode CJK, Goode AW & Scott PJ (1987) Measurement and prediction of progress in delayed wound healing. *Journal of the Royal Society of Medicine* 80: 210–212.

Centre for Health Economics (1992) *Skill Mix and the Effectiveness of Nursing Care*. University of York.

Chapman CM (1983) The paradox of nursing. *Journal of Advanced Nursing* 8: 269–272.

Chibnall JT & Tait RC (1990) The quality of life scale: a preliminary study with chronic pain patients. *Psychological Health* 4: 283–292.

Dealey C (1990) The specialist in tissue viability. *Nursing* 4(1): 16–19.

Department of Health (1993) *Clinical Audit*. London: DoH.

Donabedian A (1976) Some issues in evaluating the quality of health care. *Issues in Evaluation Research*. Kansas: American Nurses Association.

Eriksson G, Eklund AE, Torlegard K & Dauphin E (1979) Evaluation of leg ulcer treatment with stereophotogrammetry. *British Journal of Dermatology* 101: 123–131.

Fallowfield L (1990) *The Quality of Life: The Missing Dimension in Health Care*. London: Souvenir.

Fenton M (1985) Identifying competencies in the Clinical Nurse Specialist. *Journal of Nursing Administration* 15(12): 31–37.

Flanagan M (1992) The role of the specialist nurse in wound care. *Journal of Wound Care* 1(2): 45–46.

Flanagan M (1995) A contemporary approach to wound care education. *Journal of Wound Care* 4(9): 422–424.

Gwyther J (1988) Skilled dressing. *Nursing Times* 84(11): 60–61.

Hamer C, Cullum NA & Roe BH (1994) Patients' perceptions of chronic leg ulceration. *Journal of Wound Care* 3(2): 99–101.

Hamric AB & Spross JA (eds) (1989) *The Clinical Nurse Specialist in Theory and Practice*, 2nd edn. Philadelphia: WB Saunders.

Harvey G (1988) The right tools for the job. *Nursing Times* 84(26): 47–48.

Hopper A (1991) Quality assurance in outpatients departments. *Health Services Management* October, 216–218.

Humphris D (1994) *The Clinical Nurse Specialist. Issues in Practice*. London: Macmillan.

Hunt S, McKenna SP & McEwan J (1989) *The Nottingham Health Profile Users' Manual*. Manchester: Galen Research and Consultancy.

Johns C (1989) Clinical standard setting. *Surgical Nurse* June, 5–10.

Jones V (1995) Educational initiatives in wound care. *Journal of Wound Care* 4(5): 229–230.

Marr H & Giebing H (1994) *Quality Assurance in Nursing: Concepts, Methods and Case Studies*. Edinburgh: Campion.

Melhuish JM, Plassman P & Harding KG (1994) Volume and circumference of the healing wound. *Proceedings of the Third European Conference on Advances in Wound Management.* London: Macmillan.

Morison M (1992) Quality assurance and wound care. *Wound Management* 2(1): 6–7.

Plassman P & Jones BF (1992) Measuring leg ulcers by colour-coded structured light. *Journal of Wound Care* 1(3): 35–38.

Price PE & Harding KG (1993) Defining quality of life. *Journal of Wound Care* 2(5): 304–306.

Price PE, Butterworth RJ, Bale S & Harding KG (1994) Measuring quality of life in patients with granulating wounds. *Journal of Wound Care* 3(1): 49–50.

Resch CS, Kerner E, Robson MC *et al* (1988) Pressure sore volume measurement. *Journal of the American Geriatric Society* 36(5): 444–446.

Russell IT & Grimshaw JM (1992) The effectiveness of referral guidelines: a review of methods and findings of published evaluations. In: Roland MO & Coulter A (eds) *Hospital Referrals.* Oxford University Press.

Sparacino P (1986) The Clinical Nurse Specialist. *Nursing Practitioner* 1(4): 215–228.

Storr G (1988) The Clinical Nurse Specialist: from the outside looking in. *Journal of Advanced Nursing* 13: 265–272.

Todd C (1992) Quality of life and diabetes audit. *Health Psychology Update* 11: 9–14.

Wade B & Moyer A (1989) An evaluation of clinical nurse specialists. Implications for education and the organisation of care. *Senior Nurse* 9(9): 11–16.

Wallymahmed ME, Baker GA & Macfarlane IA (1991) Quality of life assessment in diabetes: a preliminary study of young adults in Liverpool. *Practical Diabetes* 9: 193–195.

Walsh M & Ford P (1989) *Nursing: Rituals, Research and Rational Actions.* London: Heinemann.

Wright CC & Whittington D (1992) *Quality Assurance — An Introduction for Health Care Professionals.* Edinburgh: Churchill Livingstone.

Appendix
Guidelines for Acute
Wound Management*

Wound Aetiology Surgical wounds are formed from incisions which are usually performed in a sterile field.

The principal purpose is to obtain access to the operative site, with minimal tissue damage.

Usually these wounds are closed by sutures and healing occurs by primary intention.

Open wounds heal by secondary intention.

Infection is the most common cause of surgical wound failure. This may be due to a number of factors, e.g.:

a) Reason for operation e.g., operating in a septic field such as a perforated appendix carries a greater risk of wound contamination

b) Type of procedure performed — knowledge of this can give an indication of probable infection organisms.

Where there is established sepsis wounds are often left open to heal by secondary intention to reduce the incidence of wound infection.

Aims of Management

- Appropriate surgery to eradicate disease process
i) Expected outcomes
- As good a cosmetic result as can be obtained
- Avoidance of excessive or persistent pain
- Avoidance of complications of surgery, e.g. wound infection, wound dehiscence
- Return patient to normal lifestyle within acceptable time scale
ii) Healing times
a) Healing by primary intention
- Acute surgical wounds should heal uneventfully within an expected time frame

* Reproduced with permission from Wound Healing Research Unit (1994) *Wound Management, Good Practice Guidance*, NHS, Cymru, Wales. Publication of these guidelines are now available from *Journal of Wound Care*, Macmillan.

b) Healing by secondary intention

■ Healing times for wounds can be predicted according to wound size.

Assessment and Diagnosis

Using the wound healing matrix the surgical wound can be assessed with particular attention to the following:

a) Type of operation/procedure

b) Appearance of wound for stage of healing

c) Type of sutures

Management/ Rationale of Care/ Treatment

i) Environment for healing

Infection Control

Infection continues to be the commonest cause of post-operative complications.

The incidence has been shown to vary between 3.5% to as high as 12.8%, depending on the type of surgery.

Patients undergoing abdominal surgery have on average a 5% rate.

The incidence of infection is raised when a wound drain is in situ.

For those wounds not contaminated during surgery, post-operative care should prevent at all costs the development of secondary infection through cross-infection.

■ Wounds should be left undisturbed unless there are visible signs of infection

■ Ritualistic daily dressing procedures should be discouraged

■ Routine use of antiseptics to clean the wound are ineffective

■ Dressing procedures should observe strict principles of asepsis

■ Communal use of dressing equipment, e.g. scissors, tapes should be avoided

■ Patients with wound infections, where possible, should be nursed separately

■ *The single most important factor in prevention of cross infection is hand disinfection following every patient contact*

Complications of surgery

Early recognition of developing complications can prevent protracted hospitalization and wound breakdown.

If abnormal picture present:

■ Observe patient and wound for early signs of clinical infection

- Observe wound daily for abnormal swelling, discolouration and formation of haematoma
- Observe for serous or sanguineous discharge

Wound dehiscence is a surgical emergency which is predisposed by chronic cough, infection and haematoma formation/wound tension. Increased tension in the wound causes reduction in blood flow and consequently hypoxia, thus causing tissue death.

ii)   Principles and methods of cleansing

Primary intention:

- Wounds healing by primary intention rarely need cleansing
- Wound dressings should not be disturbed as this causes entry of bacteria and removal of epithelium
- Wound cleansing, if required, should be performed with sodium chloride using strict asepsis

iii)   Dressings
Primary intention:

Wounds will be covered with a semipermeable film dressing immediately following surgery.

If there are no complications this dressing may be left intact until removal of sutures/clips

Secondary intention:

- Open granulating wounds are often colonized by commensals. Studies on pilonidal sinus excision wounds and abdominal wounds demonstrate the presence of bacteria, but they do not cause problems nor delay healing in all cases
- Wounds may be cleansed by allowing patients to bath or preferably shower
- Caution must be exerted to avoid cross-contamination if numerous patients are using same bathing facilities
- Community patients may care for their own wounds by showering and/ or bathing

Wounds healing by secondary intention are left open to heal by granulation. The guide for dressing criteria should be followed.

Suture removal

Suture removal is dependent upon several factors, and therefore the practitioner can only follow general guidelines.

The length of time sutures should be left is dependent upon:

- Site of the wound
- Amount of blood supply to the area
- Amount of tension and friction the wound is under
- Age and general condition of the patient

The following guide is suggested:

Head/neck   — 4–5 days
Upper limbs   — 7 days
Trunk/abdomen   — 10 days
Lower limbs   — 14 days

If the wound gapes on removal of some sutures, alternate sutures should be removed only.

In continuous sutures the wound should be reapposed with paper sutures (Steristrips) and the surgeon informed.

Sutures that are left in place too long may cause excess scarring and/or become a focus for infection causing a stitch abscess or sinus.

Evaluation Care/ Patient Outcomes

Wounds that are healing by secondary intention should have linear measurement of length, breadth and depth, on a weekly basis.

These measurements should be recorded and used in evaluating the wound's progress.

Until recently wound volume has been difficult to assess, although there is some preliminary work in this area.

Preventative Measures/Health Education

Most surgical interventions are probably unavoidable. There may be some areas where secondary prevention can help reduce the complications of surgery and lead to an improved post-operative recovery.

a) **Surgical procedure**
   Pre-op:

- Reduce length of pre-operative in-patient stay
- Avoid unnecessary skin preparation (shaving/bathing)
- Use adequate bowel preparation prior to elective surgery where appropriate

   During op:

- Avoidance of excess and rough handling of tissue/organs
- Limited use of diathermy
- Routine use of prophylactic antibiotics when indicated

- No breach of aseptic technique
- Choose appropriate suture material for type of tissue
- Limit use of wound drains with preference given to closed type drains

  Post-op:

- Prevent hypoxia and hypotension

b) **Patient preparation**

Studies have demonstrated that pre-operative information and counselling have a beneficial effect on post-operative recovery.

Information reduces anxiety levels and post-operative pain. This in turn leads to quicker mobilization and decreases the complications of surgery.

Glossary

Abscess	a collection of pus which has localized. It is formed by the liquefactive disintegration of tissue and a large accumulation of polymorphonuclear leucocytes
Albumin	a water-soluble protein. Serum albumin is the chief protein of blood plasma. It is formed principally in the liver and makes up about four-sevenths of the 6–8% protein concentration in the plasma
Alginates	a group of wound dressings derived from seaweed
Anaerobic bacteria	bacteria which thrive in an anoxic environment
Angiogenesis	the process of new blood vessel formation
Antibiotic	a chemical substance that is able to kill or inhibit the growth of micro-organisms. Antibiotics are classified according to their action on the micro-organism
Arteriosclerosis	a group of diseases characterized by thickening and loss of the elasticity of the arterial walls
Aseptic technique	a method of carrying out sterile procedures so that there is the minimum risk of introducing infection. Achieved by the sterility of equipment and a non-touch method
Autolysis	the breakdown of devitalized tissues. The disintegration of cells or tissues by endogenous enzymes
Bacteria	any prokaryotic organism. These are single-celled micro-organisms which lack a true nucleus and organelles. A single loop of double-stranded DNA makes up their genetic material
Callus	localized hyperplasia of the horny layer of the epidermis which is caused by friction or pressure
Cauterization	the application of heat sufficient to scar tissue; used to obtain haemostasis
Cellulitis	inflammation of the subcutaneous tissues. It is characterized by oedema, redness, pain and loss of function
Collagen	the main protein consitituent of white fibrous tissue (skin, bone, tendon, cartilage and connective tissue). It is composed of bundles of tropocollagen molecules, which contain three intertwined polypeptide chains
Colonization	the presence of commensal or pathogenic organisms

	which multiply on the wound but do not cause infection
Contractures	abnormal shortening of muscle or scar tissue rendering the muscle highly resistant to stretching. A contracture can lead to permanent disability
Debridement	the removal of foreign matter or devitalized, injured, infected tissue from a wound until the surrounding healthy tissue is exposed
Dehiscence	a splitting open or separation of the layers of a surgically closed wound
Devitalized	devoid of vitality or life; dead
Doppler ultrasonography	a method of measuring blood flow in peripheral arteries. Changes in blood flow may be correlated with pressure gradients across stenosed vessels and valves and can give an indication of blood supply to the distal tissues
Epithelialization	the growth of epithelium over a denuded wound surface
Endothelium	the layer of epithelial cells that line the cavities of the heart and of the blood and lymph vessels and of the serous cavities of the body
Eschar	dead, devitalized tissue
Extravasation	a discharge or escape of blood or fluid from a vessel in the tissues. Commonly associated with intravenous infusions
Exudate	wound fluid with a high content of protein and cells that has escaped from blood vessels
Fibroblast	an immature collagen producing cell of connective tissue
Fungate	to produce fungus-like growths; to grow rapidly
Granulation tissue	the new tissue formed during the proliferative phase of wound healing. It consists of connective tissue cells and ingrowing young vessels which form a cicatrix
Haematoma	a localized collection of blood which can form in an organ, space or tissue
Haemostasis	the process of stopping bleeding which can occur naturally by clot formation and artificially by compression or suturing
Hydrocolloid	a dressing material made up of a colloid in which water is the dispersion medium
Hydrogel	a dressing material which consists of a water-containing gel
Hypergranulation/ outgranulation	exhuberent amounts of soft, oedematous granulation tissue developing during healing

Hypertrophic	an increase in volume of tissue produced by enlargement of existing cells
Infection	the invasion and multiplication of micro-organisms in body fluids or tissues. The spectrum of infection agents continually changes as bacteria and viruses are capable of rapid mutation
Inflammation	the initial response to tissue injury. The inflammatory response can be caused by physical, chemical and biological agents
Ischaemia	the deficiency in blood supply to a part of the body due to functional constriction or actual obstruction of a blood vessel
Keloid	a type of scar which is often red and prominent. It is caused by excessive collagen formation in the corium during connective tissue repair
Keratin	an insoluble protein forming the principal component of epidermis, hair, nails and tooth enamel
Leucocytes	the colourless blood corpuscles whose chief function is to protect the body against micro-organisms
Lymphocyte	a mononuclear, non-granular leucocyte, chiefly a product of lymphoid tissue, which participates in the immune response
Maceration	excessive moisture and redness in the tissues surrounding a wound edge
Macrophage	any of the large, mononuclear, phagocytotic cells derived from monocytes that are found in the walls of blood vessels and in loose connective tissue. They become stimulated by inflammation on initial angiogenesis
Matrix	the intracellular substance of a tissue which forms the framework of tissues
Maturation	a phase in wound healing where scar tissue is remodelled
Myofibroblast	a differentiated fibroblast containing the ultrastructural features of a fibroblast and a smooth muscle cell and containing many actin-rich microfilaments
Necrosis/ nectrotic tissue	the death of previously viable tissue
Proliferation	the growth or reproduction of tissue as part of the healing process
Proline	a cyclic amino acid occurring in proteins; it is a major constituent of collagen
Pus	a protein-rich liquid which consists of exudate, dead macrophages and bacteria

Scab	the dry crust forming over an open wound which consists of skin and debris
Septicaemia	blood poisoning, a systemic disease where pathogenic micro-organisms are present and multiply in the blood. A life-threatening disease
Slough	a mass of dead tissue in or cast out of living tissue
Suppuration	formation of discharge or pus
Suture	a stitch or series of stitches made to secure opposition of the edges of a surgical or traumatic wound

Specialist Journals and Useful Address

Relevant Specialist Journals

Advances in Wound Care (USA)
Diabetes, American Diabetes Association, USA
Elderly Care, RCN Publishing Ltd, bi-monthly
Journal of Enterostomal Therapy (USA)
Journal of Tissue Viability, Tissue Viability Society, quarterly
Journal of Wound Care, Macmillan Magazines, bi-monthly
Nursing Journal of the Tissue Viability Society, supplement in Nursing Standard
Wounds (USA)
Primary Health Care, RCN Publishing, bi-monthly
Primary Intention, Australia
Surgical Nurse, The Medicine Group Ltd
Wound Care, in Association with the Wound Care Society, quarterly supplement in Nursing Times
Wound Management, Media Medica. Quarterly

Specialist Wound Care Organizations

European Tissue Repair Society,
Dr G Cherry,
Wound Healing Institute,
Churchills Hospital,
Headington,
Oxford OX3 7LJ

European Wound Management
Association,
PO Box 864,
London SE1 8TT

Tissue Viability Society,
Wessex Rehabilitation Unit,
Odstock Hospital,
Salisbury,
Wiltshire

Venous Forum,
C Richard Corbett,
Hon Sec: Venous Forum of the
Royal Society of Medicine,
The Ashdown Hospital,
Burrell Road,
Haywards Heath,
West Sussex RH16 1UD

Wound Care Society,
PO Box 263,
Northampton NN3 4US

Wound Healing Society,
Headquarters,
NIS Travel/WHS,
7270 Metro Boulevard,
Minneapolis,
MN 55439, USA

Other Useful Addresses

Age Concern England (National
Old Peoples' Welfare Council),
60 Pitcairn Road,
Mitcham,
Surrey CR4 3LL

APEX Partnership,
22–24 Worple Road,
Wimbledon,
London SW19 4DD

Association of British Paediatric
Nurses (ABPN),
PO Box 14,
Ashton-under-Lyne OL5 9HH

Association of Community Health
Councils for England and Wales,
30 Drayton Park,
London N5 1PB

Association of Radical Midwives,
c/o Haringey Women's Centre,
40 Turnpike Lane,
London N8

Breast Care and Mastectomy
Association,
26a Harrison Street,
London WC1H 8JG

BRIDGES,
Greytree Lodge,
Second Avenue,
Ross-on-Wye,
Herefordshire HR9 7HT

British Diabetic Association,
10 Queen Anne Street,
London W1M 0BD

British Dietetic Association,
Daimler House,
Paradise Circus,
Queensway,
Birmingham B1 2BJ

British Medical Association,
BMA House,
Tavistock Square,
London WC1H 9JP

Cancer Link,
17 Britannia Street,
London WC1X 9JN

Carer's National Association,
29 Chilwalk Mews,
London W2 3RG

Centre for Health Economics,
University of York,
Heslington,
York YO1 5DD

Community Health UK (National
Community Health Resource),
6 Terrace Walk,
Bath,
Avon BA1 1LN

Department of Health,
Alexander Fleming House,
Elephant and Castle,
London SE1 6BY

ENB Careers,
PO Box 356,
Sheffield S8 0SJ

English National Board for Nursing,
Midwifery and Health Visiting
(ENB),
Victory House,
170 Tottenham Court Road,
London W1P 0HA

Gerontology Nutrition Unit,
Royal Free Hospital,
School of Medicine,
21 Pond Street,
London NW3 2PN

Health Education Authority,
Hamilton House,
Mabledon Place,
London WC1H 9TX

Health Education Authority,
78 New Oxford Street,
London WC1A 1AH

Help the Aged,
16–18 St James's Walk,
London EC1R 0BE

Home from Hospital (HFH),
20 Westfield Road,
Edgbaston,
Birmingham B15 3QG

Hospice Information Service,
St Christopher's Hospice,
51–59 Lawrie Park Road,
Sydenham,
London SE26 6DZ

Infection Control Nurses
Association (ICNA),
c/o Janet Roberts,
Clatterbridge Hospital,
Bebington,
Wirral,
Merseyside L63 4JY

Institute of Health Education (IHE),
14 High Elm Road,
Hale Barns,
Altrincham,
Cheshire WA15 0HS

Institution of Environmental Health
Officers,
Chadwick Court,
15 Hatfields,
London SE1 8DJ

King's Fund Centre,
126 Albert Street,
London NW1 7NF

King's Medical Research Trust,
Rayne Institute,
123 Coldharbour Lane,
London SE5 9NU

MacMillan Cancer Relief,
Anchor House,
15–19 Britten Street,
London SW3 3TY

Malcolm Sargent Cancer Fund for
Children,
14 Abingdon Road,
London W8 6AF

Marie Curie Memorial Foundation,
28 Belgrave Square,
London SW1X 8QG

National Association of Health
Authorities and Trusts,
Birmingham Research Park,
Vincent Drive,
Edgbaston,
Birmingham B15 2SQ

National Board for Nursing,
Midwifery and Health Visiting for
Northern Ireland,
123/137 York Street,
Belfast BT15 1JB

National Board for Nursing,
Midwifery and Health Visiting for
Scotland,
Trinity Park House,
South Trinity Road,
Edinburgh EH5 3SF

National Society for the Prevention
of Cruelty to Children (NSPCC),
67 Saffron Hill,
London EC1N 8RS

Parent's Friend,
c/o Voluntary Action Leeds,
Stringer House,
34 Lupton Street,
Hunslet,
Leeds LS10 2QW

Royal College of Nursing and
Council of Nurses of the United
Kingdom,
20 Cavendish Square,
London W1N 0AB

Royal Institute of Public Health and
Hygiene,
28 Portland Place,
London W1N 4DE

Royal National Pension Fund for
Nurses,
Burdett House,
15 Buckingham Street,
Strand,
London WC2N 6ED

Royal Society for the Prevention of
Accidents (RoSPA),
Cannon House,
The Priory,
Queensway,
Birmingham B4 6BS

Royal Society of Medicine,
1 Wimpole Street,
London W1M 8AE

UNISON (formerly COHSE,
NUPE and NALGO),
UNISON Towers,
137 High Holborn,
London WC1

United Kingdom Central Council
for Nursing,
Midwifery and Health Visiting
(UKCC),
23 Portland Place,
London W1N 3AF

Welsh National Board for Nursing,
Midwifery and Health Visiting,
13th Floor,
Pearl Assurance House,
Greyfriars Road,
Cardiff CF1 3AG

INDEX